The Future *of* Public Health

Committee for the
Study of the Future of Public Health
Division of Health Care Services
Institute of Medicine

NATIONAL ACADEMY PRESS
Washington, D.C.   1988

NATIONAL ACADEMY PRESS ● 2101 Constitution Ave., NW ● Washington, DC 20418

NOTICE: The project that is the subject of this report was approved by the Governing Board of the National Research Council, whose members are drawn from the councils of the National Academy of Sciences, the National Academy of Engineering, and the Institute of Medicine. The members of the committee responsible for the report were chosen for their special competences and with regard for appropriate balance.

This report has been reviewed by a group other than the authors according to procedures approved by a Report Review Committee consisting of members of the National Academy of Sciences, the National Academy of Engineering, and the Institute of Medicine.

The Institute of Medicine was chartered in 1970 by the National Academy of Sciences to enlist distinguished members of the appropriate professions in the examination of policy matters pertaining to the health of the public. In this, the Institute acts under both the Academy's 1863 congressional charter responsibility to be an adviser to the federal government and its own initiative in identifying issues of medical care, research, and education.

This project was supported by the W. K. Kellogg Foundation and two agencies of the U.S. Public Health Service (the Centers for Disease Control and the Health Resources and Services Administration, Contract No.U50/CCU 300989-01).

Library of Congress Cataloging-in-Publication Data

Institute of Medicine (U.S.). Committee for the Study of the Future of Public Health.
    The future of public health/Committee for the Study of the Future of Public Health, Division of Health Care Services, Institute of Medicine.
      p. cm.—(Publication IOM; 88-02)
    Includes bibliography and index.
    ISBN 0-309-03830-8 (paper); ISBN 0-309-03831-6 (cloth)
    1. Public health—Forecasting—United States.   I. Title.
II. Series: IOM publication; 88-02.
    [DNLM: 1. Health Services—United States.   2. Public Health—history—United States.   3. Public Health—trends—United States.
4. Quality of Health Care—United States.   W 84 AA1 I482f]
RA445.I57 1988
362.1′0973—dc19
DNLM/DLC
for Library of Congress
    88-25538
    CIP

First Printing, October 1988
Second Printing, February 1989
Third Printing, April 1989
Fourth Printing, July 1989
Fifth Printing, January 1990

Committee for the
Study of the Future of Public Health

Preface

In recent years, there has been a growing sense that public health, as a profession, as a governmental activity, and as a commitment of society is neither clearly defined, adequately supported, nor fully understood. Concerns for chronic diseases, geriatric disorders, substance abuse, teen pregnancy, and toxic substances in the environment seem to some critics of public health, both within and outside government, to be inadequately addressed by a public health apparatus originally conceived and constructed to meet a different set of concerns. To many observers, problems of delivery, financing, coverage, and quality of personal health services seem inadequately addressed by health departments and other official agencies.

Yet, many of these critics express the belief that the health problems now facing the public are complex, challenging, and diverse; that they cover a broad spectrum of infectious and chronic diseases; that they demand superior personal and environmental health services; and that they involve preventive, therapeutic, and rehabilitative intervention. This very complexity, when added to the perceived potential vulnerability to new epidemics and environmental hazards of virtually the entire population, lead many observers to conclude that a governmental presence, perhaps an expanded presence, in health has never been more necessary.

But what is the most appropriate nature of that governmental presence? How should government's role relate to that of the private sector? How should governmental responsibility for public health be apportioned among local, state, and federal levels? Should government be the health care provider of last resort or does it have a greater responsibility? Should public health consist only of a necessary residuum of activities not met by private providers? How should governmental activities directed toward the maintenance of an environment conductive to health be apportioned among various agencies? But above all, just what is public health? What does it include and what does it exclude? Based on an appropriate definition, what kinds of programs and agencies should be constructed to meet the needs and demands of the public, which is often resistant to an increasing role, or at least an increasing cost, of government?

All these questions and more are considered in this report. Its recommendations and conclusions are based on an extensive contemporary assessment of public health as it is now practiced, as well as the opinions of hundreds of individual commentators. But ultimately, when data gathering has been completed, a synthesis and integration of findings must occur. It is this synthesis that has led to the results reported here. It is the hope of the committee, staff, reviewers, the Institute of Medicine, and the sponsors that this report will be helpful in focusing attention upon the public health and some means for its advancement.

RICHARD D. REMINGTON,
Chairman, Committee for the
Study of the Future of Public Health

To Beverlee A. Myers

Beverlee Myers was a member of this committee until her untimely death in December 1986. Her contributions to the formulation and early implementation of the committee's work were extraordinary, even after her final illness was advanced. These contributions reflected her characteristic insight, energy, and dedication to public health. Her remarkable ability to dissect and analyze complex issues, and the coupling of that analysis with her broad experience in public health activities, enabled all of us to see our task more clearly. She was an exemplar of the best in public service. We share with many an appreciation of her accomplishments and a deep sense of loss. We dedicate this report to the memory of Beverlee Myers with affection and respect.

Acknowledgments

The committee thanks the many persons who assisted in the conduct of this study. Without their contributions, the study could not have been accomplished.

First, it thanks the practitioners of public health who shared their time and knowledge. Special thanks go to the several hundred people who welcomed the committee into their communities in the six states it visited. The persons with whom the committee spoke in California, Mississippi, New Jersey, South Dakota, Washington, and West Virginia were gracious, thoughtful, and informative beyond request. Many spent hours patiently explaining public health issues and operations within their communities; others spent considerable time assisting with arrangements for the visits. The insights and information they provided are an important foundation of this report. Another several hundred people from dozens of states spoke at four public meetings. The committee thanks them for their words and thoughts. And the committee thanks the health officials of Toronto, Canada, who provided valuable information on the Canadian public health system. We also thank the many public health educators, public health practitioners, and others concerned with public health who participated in the conference on education and training for public health in Houston, Texas, in March 1987.

The staffs of numerous national organizations, including the Public Health Foundation, the Association of State and Territorial Health Officials, the Association of Schools of Public Health, the American Public Health Association, and others provided assistance, advice, and information crucial to the report. And the staff of the Health Sciences Center of the University of Texas at Houston School of Public Health assisted in sponsoring the conference on research, education, and training in public health. The staffs of the organizations sponsoring the report—the Kellogg Foundation, the Centers for Disease Control, and the Health Resources and Services Administration—were also unfailingly encouraging and generous with information and assistance.

An additional person must also be thanked for finding and returning notes and drafts that were lost when baggage was stolen at the airport. The committee is grateful to him for his public spirit at a crucial stage in the preparation of the report. Without his assistance, completion of the report would have been considerably more difficult.

The committee would also like to thank its staff. Karl Yordy, Study Director, Camilla Stivers, Associate Study Director, Susan Sherman, Research Associate, and H. Donald Tiller, Administrative Secretary, served with grace, insight, and exceptional diligence in carrying out the complex arrangements for this study and in pursuing the suggestions of the committee.

Finally, the committee would like to state its great gratitude and admiration for the hundreds of people with whom it spoke who have dedicated their lives to protecting the public's health. Without the unflagging commitment of these people, the nation's public health system would not be as successful as it is. While the committee presents many suggestions for improving the public health system in the following report, it is confident that improvements can be made precisely because the individuals who work in the system are so capable. The committee wishes to thank these individuals for their tireless contributions to society.

Contents

APPENDIXES

The
Future
of
Public Health

Summary and Recommendations

WHY STUDY PUBLIC HEALTH

Many of the major improvements in the health of the American people have been accomplished through public health measures. Control of epidemic diseases, safe food and water, and maternal and child health services are only a few of the public health achievements that have prevented countless deaths and improved the quality of American life. But the public has come to take the success of public health for granted. Health officials have difficulty communicating a sense of urgency about the need to maintain current preventive efforts and to sustain the capability to meet future threats to the public's health.

This study was undertaken to address a growing perception among the Institute of Medicine membership and others concerned with the health of the public that this nation has lost sight of its public health goals and has allowed the system of public health activities to fall into disarray. Public health is what we, as a society, do collectively to assure the conditions in which people can be healthy. This requires that continuing and emerging threats to the health of the public be successfully countered. These threats include immediate crises, such as the AIDS epidemic; enduring problems, such as injuries and chronic illness; and impending crises foreshadowed by such developments as the toxic by-products of a modern economy.

These and many other problems demonstrate the need to protect the nation's health through effective, organized, and sustained efforts by the public sector. Unfortunately, the findings of this committee confirm the concerns that led to the study. The current state of our abilities for effective public health action, as documented in this volume, is cause for national concern and for the development of a plan of action for needed improvements. In the committee's view, we have slackened our public health vigilance nationally, and the health of the public is unnecessarily threatened as a result.

An impossible responsibility has been placed on America's public health agencies: to serve as stewards of the basic health needs of entire populations, but at the same time avert impending disasters and provide personal health care to those rejected by the rest of the health system. The wonder is not that American public health has problems, but that so much has been done so well, and with so little.

The Committee for the Study of the Future of Public Health is keenly aware of the public health system's many achievements and of the dedication and sustained efforts of public health workers across the country. The committee's purpose, however, is to bring the difficulties of public health to the attention of the nation in order to mobilize action to strengthen public health. Successes as great as those of the past are still possible, but not without public concern and concerted action to restore America's public health capacity.

This volume envisions the future of public health, analyzes the current situation and how it developed, and presents a plan of action that will, in the committee's judgment, provide a solid foundation for a strong public health capability throughout the nation.

THE APPROACH

During the past 2 years, the committee has studied America's public health system in detail. It has attempted to see public health in action, as revealed by data and as perceived by those involved in it, both inside and outside public health agencies. It has examined demographic and epidemiologic statistics, agency budgets, organization charts, program plans, statutes, and regulations. It has visited localities in six states and spoken with more than 350 people: state and local health officers, public health nurses, sanitarians, legislators, citizen activists, public administrators, voluntary agency personnel, private physicians, and many others. In addition, public meetings were held in Boston, Chicago, New Orleans, and Las Vegas, as well as a conference in Houston on public health education attended by public health educators and practitioners. Finally, the committee reviewed the history of American public health and visited with health officials in Toronto to glimpse the enterprise as practiced in another country, where universal entitlement to medical care is part of the context for that practice.

THE STATE OF U.S. PUBLIC HEALTH

Throughout the history of public health, two major factors have determined how problems were solved: the level of scientific and technical knowledge, and the content of public values and popular opinions. Over time, public health measures have changed with important advances in understanding the causes and control of disease. In addition, practice was affected by popular beliefs about illness and by public views on appropriate governmental action. As poverty and disease came to be seen as societal as well as personal problems, and as governmental involvement in societal concerns increased, collective action against disease was gradually accepted. Health became a social as well as individual responsibility. At the same time, advances such as the discovery of bacteria and identification of better ways to control and prevent communicable disease made possible effective community action under the auspices of increasingly professional public health agencies.

THE PUBLIC HEALTH MISSION

Knowledge and values today remain decisive elements in the shaping of public health practice. But they blend less harmoniously than they once did. On the surface there appears to be widespread agreement on the overall mission of public health, as reflected in such comments to the committee as "public health does things that benefit everybody," or "public health prevents illness and educates the population." But when it comes to translating broad statements into effective action, little consensus can be found. Neither among the providers nor the beneficiaries of public health programs is there a shared sense of what the citizenry should expect in the way of services, and both the mix and the intensity of services vary widely from place to place.

In one state the committee visited, the state health department was a major provider of prenatal care for poor women; in other places, women who could not pay got no care. Some state health departments are active and well equipped, while others perform fewer functions and get by on relatively meager resources. Localities vary even more widely: in some places, the local health departments are larger and more sophisticated technically than many state health departments. But in too many localities, there is no health department. Perhaps the area is visited occasionally by a "circuit-riding" public health nurse—and perhaps not.

Lack of agreement about the public health mission is also reflected in the diversion in some states of traditional public health functions, such as water and air pollution control, to separate departments of environmental services, where the health effects of pollutants often receive less notice.

In some states, mental health is seen as a public health responsibility, but in many the two are organizationally distinct, making it difficult to coordinate services to multiproblem clients. Some health departments are part of larger departments of "social and health services," where public health scientists find their approaches, which benefit society as a whole, stamped with a negative welfare label.

Such extreme variety of available services and organizational arrangements suggests that contemporary public health is defined less by what public health professionals know how to do than by what the political system in a given area decides is appropriate or feasible.

PROFESSIONAL EXPERTISE AND THE POLITICAL PROCESS

Tension between professional expertise and politics can be observed throughout the nation's public health system. Public health professionals rely on expert knowledge derived from such areas as epidemiology and biostatistics to identify and deal with the health needs of whole populations. A central tenet of their professional ethic is commitment to use this knowledge to fulfill the public interest in reducing human suffering and enhancing the quality of life. Thus their aim is to maximize the influence of accurate data and professional judgment on decision-making—to make decisions as comprehensive and objective as possible.

The dynamics of American politics, however, make it difficult to fulfill this commitment. Decision-making in public health, as in other areas, is driven by crises, hot issues, and the concerns of organized interest groups. Decisions are made largely on the basis of competition, bargaining, and influence rather than comprehensive analysis. The idea that politics can be restricted to the legislative arena, while the work of public agencies remains neutral and expert, has been discredited. Professional analysis and judgment must compete with other perspectives for policy attention and support.

Public health has had great difficulty accommodating itself to these political dynamics. Technical knowledge in fact plays a much more restricted role in public health decision-making than it once did, despite the fact that we now know more. The impact of politics is clearly evident in the rapid turnover among public health officials (the average tenure of a state health officer is now only 2 years); in a marked shift toward political appointees as opposed to career professionals in the top ranks of health agencies; and in the gradual disappearance of state boards of health, which have dwindled by half (from nearly all states to 24) in only 25 years. Too frequently during its investigations, the committee heard legislators and members of the general public castigate public health professionals as paper-shufflers, out of touch with reality, and caught up in red tape. There is a sharp tendency to take what are perceived as "important" programs (for example, Medicaid and environmental programs) away from health departments. The growing perception of health as big business has led to attempts to take public health "out of the hands of the doctors" by interposing a nonmedical administrator between the health officer and elected officials.

Perhaps because they view their professional knowledge and skills as effective and therefore obviously valuable, public health professionals appear to have been slow in developing strategies to demonstrate the worth of their efforts to legislators and the public. Public health crises, not public health successes, make headlines. A number of well-informed members of the public had only vague ideas about what their local health department did. Without broad support, public health officials appear defensive and self-serving when they attempt to answer the criticisms of legislators or mobilize needed resources. Yet many public health professionals who talked with us seemed to regard politics as a contaminant of an ideally rational decision-making process rather than as an essential element of democratic governance. We saw much evidence of isolation and little evidence of constituency building, citizen participation, or continuing (as opposed to crisis-driven) communications with elected officials or with the community at large.

PUBLIC HEALTH AND THE MEDICAL PROFESSION

The political difficulties of public health are reflected in an especially vivid way in its associations with private medicine. Historically, this has been an uneasy relationship. The discovery of bacteria, which proved such a boon to public health's disease control efforts, also brought it into competition with physicians, inasmuch as control measures such as immunizations were carried out not in the environment but on individual patients, who were the purview of the private doctor. Today, while numerous examples can be found of medical community support for public health activities (witness the American Medical Association's stance on AIDS), too often confrontation and suspicion are evident on both sides. For example, the director of one state medical association characterized the health department as distrustful of physicians and cited the director's effort to push a mandatory data-reporting system through the legislature without consulting the society. The committee found medical leaders who were unaware of public health activities in their communities; yet these same leaders are crucial to the implementation of many public health measures and vital in building political support.

THE KNOWLEDGE BASE AND ITS APPLICATION

This summary of the state of U.S. public health began with the observation that both technical knowledge and public values determine how public health is practiced. Clearly, the current impact of public values is troublesome, as political dilemmas attest. But there are also problems on the knowledge front.

Effective public health action must be based on accurate knowledge of the causes and distribution of health problems and of effective interventions. Despite much progress, there are still significant knowledge gaps for many public health problems, for example, the health risks of long-term exposure to certain toxic chemicals or the role of stress in disease.

Because public health is an applied activity, operating under fiscal constraints, it is often difficult to mobilize and sustain necessary research. In our site visits, we found that only one of six states had made a substantial investment in research. Similarly, technical expertise is unevenly distributed: public health employees in some larger states have a considerable skill level, but many others do not. The problem is exacerbated by a shortage of epidemiologists and other trained experts. In many jurisdictions low salary structures and unrewarding professional environments may further inhibit the acquisition of expertise.

In addition, there has been little attention in public health to management as a technical skill in its own right. Management of a public health agency is a demanding, high-visibility assignment requiring, in addition to technical and political acumen, the ability to motivate and lead personnel, to plan and allocate agency resources, and to sense and deal with changes in the agency's environment and to relate the agency to the larger community. Progress in public health in the United States has been greatly advanced throughout its history by outstanding individuals who fortuitously combined all these qualities. Today, the need for leaders is too great to leave their emergence to chance. Yet there is little specific focus in public health education on leadership development, and low salaries and a low public image make it difficult to attract outstanding people into the profession and to retain them until they are ready for top posts.

THE FUTURE OF PUBLIC HEALTH: RECOMMENDATIONS

In conducting this study, the committee has sought to take a fresh look at public health—its mission, its current state, and the barriers to improvement. The committee has concluded that effective public health activities are essential to the health and well-being of the American people, now and in the future. But public health is currently in disarray. Some of the frequently heard criticisms of public health are deserved, but this society has contributed to the disarray by lack of clarity and agreement about the mission of public health, the role of government, and the specific means necessary to accomplish public health objectives. To provide a set of directions for public health that can attract the support of the total society, the committee has made three basic recommendations dealing with:

- the mission of public health,
- the governmental role in fulfilling the mission, and
- the responsibilities unique to each level of government.

The rest of the recommendations are instrumental in implementing the basic recommendations for the future of public health. These instrumental recommendations fall into the following categories: statutory framework; structural and organizational steps; strategies to build the fundamental capacities of public health agencies—technical, political, managerial, programmatic, and fiscal; and education for public health.

THE PUBLIC HEALTH MISSION, GOVERNMENTAL ROLE, AND LEVELS OF RESPONSIBILITY

MISSION

- **The committee defines the mission of public health as fulfilling society's interest in assuring conditions in which people can be healthy.** Its aim is to generate organized community effort to address the public interest in health by applying scientific and technical knowledge to prevent disease and promote health. The mission of public health is addressed by private organizations and individuals as well as by public agencies. But the governmental public health agency has a unique function: to see to it that vital elements are in place and that the mission is adequately addressed.

THE GOVERNMENTAL ROLE IN PUBLIC HEALTH

- **The committee finds that the core functions of public health agencies at all levels of government are assessment, policy development, and assurance.**

Assessment

- **The committee recommends that every public health agency regularly and systematically collect, assemble, analyze, and make available information on the health of the community, including statistics on health status, community health needs, and epidemiologic and other studies of health problems.** Not every agency is large enough to conduct these activities directly; intergovernmental and interagency cooperation is essential. Nevertheless each agency bears the responsibility for seeing that the assessment function is fulfilled. This basic function of public health cannot be delegated.

Policy Development

• The committee recommends that every public health agency exercise its responsibility to serve the public interest in the development of comprehensive public health policies by promoting use of the scientific knowledge base in decision-making about public health and by leading in developing public health policy. Agencies must take a strategic approach, developed on the basis of a positive appreciation for the democratic political process.

Assurance

• The committee recommends that public health agencies assure their constituents that services necessary to achieve agreed upon goals are provided, either by encouraging actions by other entities (private or public sector), by requiring such action through regulation, or by providing services directly.

• The committee recommends that each public health agency involve key policymakers and the general public in determining a set of high-priority personal and communitywide health services that governments will guarantee to every member of the community. This guarantee should include subsidization or direct provision of high-priority personal health services for those unable to afford them.

LEVELS OF RESPONSIBILITY

In addition to these functions, which are common to federal, state, and local governments, each level of government has unique responsibilities.

States

• The committee believes that states are and must be the central force in public health. They bear primary public sector responsibility for health.

• The committee recommends that the public health duties of states should include the following:

—assessment of health needs in the state based on statewide data collection;

—assurance of an adequate statutory base for health activities in the state;

—establishment of statewide health objectives, delegating power to localities as appropriate and holding them accountable;

—assurance of appropriate organized statewide effort to develop and maintain essential personal, educational, and environmental health services; provision of access to necessary services; and solution of problems inimical to health;

—guarantee of a minimum set of essential health services; and

—support of local service capacity, especially when disparities in local ability to raise revenue and/or administer programs require subsidies, technical assistance, or direct action by the state to achieve adequate service levels.

Federal

• The committee recommends the following as federal public health obligations:

—support of knowledge development and dissemination through data gathering, research, and information exchange;

—establishment of nationwide health objectives and priorities, and stimulation of debate on interstate and national public health issues;

—provision of technical assistance to help states and localities determine their own objectives and to carry out action on national and regional objectives;

—provision of funds to states to strengthen state capacity for services, especially to achieve an adequate minimum capacity, and to achieve national objectives; and

—assurance of actions and services that are in the public interest of the entire nation such as control of AIDS and similar communicable diseases, interstate environmental actions, and food and drug inspection.

Localities

Because of great diversity in size, powers, and capacities of local governments, generalizations must be made with caution. Nevertheless, **no citizen from any community, no matter how small or remote, should be without identifiable and realistic access to the benefits of public health protection, which is possible only through a local component of the public health delivery system.**

• The committee recommends the following functions for local public health units:

—assessment, monitoring, and surveillance of local health problems and needs and of resources for dealing with them;

—policy development and leadership that foster local involvement and a sense of ownership, that emphasize local needs, and that advocate equitable distribution of public resources and complementary private activities commensurate with community needs; and

—assurance that high-quality services, including personal health services, needed for the protection of public health in the community are available and accessible to all persons; that the community receives proper consideration in the allocation of federal and state as well as local resources for public health; and that the community is informed about how to obtain public health, including personal health, services, or how to comply with public health requirements.

FULFILLING THE GOVERNMENT ROLE: IMPLEMENTING RECOMMENDATIONS

A number of specific steps should be taken to enable public health agencies to fulfill the functions outlined above. These include modification of public health statutes, changes in the organizational structure, special linkages, strategies for building agency capacity, and improvements in education for public health.

STATUTES

• **The committee recommends that states review their public health statutes and make revisions necessary to accomplish the following two objectives:**

—**clearly delineate the basic authority and responsibility entrusted to public health agencies, boards, and officials at the state and local levels and the relationships between them; and**

—**support a set of modern disease control measures that address contemporary health problems such as AIDS, cancer, and heart disease, and incorporate due process safeguards (notice, hearings, administrative review, right to counsel, standards of evidence).**

ORGANIZATIONAL STRUCTURE

States

As the primary locus for action in the public health arena, states must establish a clear organizational focal point for public health responsibility.

• **The committee recommends that each state have a department of health that groups all primarily health-related functions under professional direction—separate from income maintenance. Responsibilities of this department should include disease prevention and health promotion, Medicaid and other indigent health care activities, mental health and substance abuse, environmental responsibilities that clearly require health expertise, and health planning and regulation of health facilities and professions.**

• **The committee recommends that each state have a state health council that reports regularly on the health of the state's residents, makes health policy recommendations to the governor and legislature, promulgates public** health regulations, reviews the work of the state health department, and recommends candidates for director of the department.

• The committee recommends that the director of the department of health be a cabinet (or equivalent-level) officer. Ideally, the director should have doctoral-level education as a physician or in another health profession, as well as education in public health itself and extensive public sector administrative experience. Provisions for tenure in office, such as a specific term of appointment, should promote needed continuity of professional leadership.

• The committee recommends that each state establish standards for local public health functions, specifying what minimum services must be offered, by what unit of government, and how services are to be financed. States (unless providing local services directly) should hold localities accountable for these services and for addressing statewide health objectives, using the *Model Standards: A Guide for Community Preventive Health Services* as a guide.

Localities

Local circumstances will determine the appropriate balance between state and local responsibilities. But in general the committee prefers delegation of responsibilities to the local level.

• The committee finds that the larger the population served by a single multipurpose government, as well as the stronger the history of local control, the more realistic the delegation of responsibility becomes: for example, to a large metropolitan city, county, or service district. Two attributes of such a locally responsible system are strongly recommended:

—To promote clear accountability, public health responsibility should be delegated to only one unit of government in a locality. For example, in the case of large cities, public health responsibility should be lodged either in the municipal or the county government, but not both.

—Where sparse population or scarce resources prevail, delegation to regional single-purpose units, such as multicounty health districts, may be appropriate. In order to be effective, health districts must be linked by formal ties to, and receive resources from, general-purpose governments.

• The committee recommends that mechanisms be instituted to promote local accountability and assure the maintenance of adequate and equitable levels of service and qualified personnel.

• The committee finds that the need for a clear focal point at the local level is as great as at the state level, and for the same reasons. Where the scale of government activity permits, localities should establish public health councils to report to elected officials on local health needs and on the performance of the local health agency.

Federal

• The committee recommends that the federal government identify more clearly, in formal structure and actual practice, the specific officials and agencies with primary responsibility for carrying out the federal public health functions recommended earlier.

• The committee recommends the establishment of a task force to consider what structure or programmatic changes would be desirable to enhance the federal government's ability to fulfill the public health leadership responsibilities recommended in this report.

SPECIAL LINKAGES

The committee finds that environmental health and mental health activities are frequently isolated from state and local public health agencies, resulting in disjointed policy development, fragmented service delivery, lack of accountability, and a generally weakened public health effort.

Environmental Health

The removal of environmental health authority from public health agencies has led to fragmented responsibility, lack of coordination, and inadequate attention to the health dimensions of environmental problems.

• The committee recommends that state and local health agencies strengthen their capacities for identification, understanding, and control of environmental problems as health hazards. The agencies cannot simply be advocates for the health aspects of environmental issues, but must have direct operational involvement.

Mental Health

The separation of public health and mental health leads to fragmentation at the service delivery point, to the detriment of clients.

• The committee recommends that those engaged in knowledge development and policy planning in public health and in mental health, respectively, devote a specific effort to strengthening linkages with the other field, particularly in order to identify strategies to integrate these functions at the service delivery level.

• The committee recommends that a study of the public health/mental health interface be done in order to document how the lack of linkages with public health hampers the mental health mission.

Social Services

In states where public health is part of a "super" department of social services, the income maintenance function tends to detract from communitywide services and give public health a negative welfare image.

• **The committee recommends that public health be separated organizationally from income maintenance, but that public health agencies maintain close working relationships with social service agencies in order to act as effective advocates for, and to cooperate with, social service agency provision of social services that have an impact on health.**

Care of the Indigent

Many public health agencies have become last-resort providers of personal medical care, draining vital resources away from populationwide services.

• **The committee endorses the conclusion of the President's Commission for the Study of Ethical Problems in Medical Care and Biomedical and Behavioral Research that the ultimate responsibility for assuring equitable access to health care for all, through a combination of public and private sector action, rests with the federal government.**

• **The committee finds that, until adequate federal action is forthcoming, public health agencies must continue to serve, with quality and respect and to the best of their ability, the priority personal health care needs of uninsured, underinsured, and Medicaid clients.**

STRATEGIES FOR CAPACITY BUILDING

To equip public health agencies to fulfill adequately their assessment, policy development, and assurance functions, it is necessary to go beyond reorganization to build agency competence. The types of competence needed are technical, political, managerial, programmatic, and fiscal. The committee recommends the following steps.

Technical

• **A uniform national data set should be established that will permit valid comparison of local and state health data with those of the nation and of other states and localities and that will facilitate progress toward national health objectives and implementation of** *Model Standards: A Guide for Community Preventive Health Services.*

• **There should be an institutional home in each state and at the federal level for development and dissemination of knowledge, including research and** the provision of technical assistance to lower levels of government and to academic institutions and voluntary organizations.

• Research should be conducted at the federal, state, and local levels into population-based health problems, including biological, environmental, and behavioral issues. In addition to conducting research directly, the federal government should support research by states, localities, universities, and the private sector.

Political

• Public health agency leaders should develop relationships with and educate legislators and other public officials on community health needs, on public health issues, and on the rationale for strategies advocated and pursued by the health department. These relationships should be cultivated on an ongoing basis rather than being neglected until a crisis develops.

• Agencies should strengthen the competence of agency personnel in community relations and citizen participation techniques and develop procedures to build citizen participation into program implementation.

• Agencies should develop and cultivate relationships with physicians and other private sector representatives. Physicians and other health professionals are important instruments of public health by virtue of such activities as counseling patients on health promotion and providing immunizations. They are important determinants of public attitudes and of the image of public health. Public health leaders should take the initiative to seek working relationships and support among local, state, and national medical and other professional societies and academic medical centers.

• Agencies should seek stronger relationships and common cause with other professional and citizen groups pursuing interests with health implications, including voluntary health organizations, groups concerned with improving social services or the environment, and groups concerned with economic development.

• Agencies should undertake education of the public on community health needs and public health policy issues.

• Agencies should review the quality of "street-level" contacts between department employees and clients, and where necessary conduct in-service training to ensure that members of the public are treated with cordiality and respect.

Managerial

• Greater emphasis in public health curricula should be placed on managerial and leadership skills, such as the ability to communicate important agency values to employees and enlist their commitment; to sense and deal with important changes in the environment; to plan, mobilize, and use resources effectively; and to relate the operation of the agency to its larger community role.

• Demonstrated management competence as well as technical/professional skills should be a requirement for upper-level management posts.

• Salaries and benefits should be improved for health department managers, especially health officers, and systems should be instituted so that they can carry retirement benefits with them when they move among different levels and jurisdictions of government.

Programmatic

• The committee recommends that public health professionals place more emphasis on factors that influence health-related behavior and develop comprehensive strategies that take these factors into account.

Fiscal

• The committee recommends the following policies with respect to intergovernmental strategies for strengthening the fiscal base of public health:

—Federal support of state-level health programs should help balance disparities in revenue-generating capacities and encourage state attention to national health objectives. Particular vehicles for such support should include "core" funding with appropriate accountability mechanisms, as well as funds targeted for specific uses.

—State support of local-level health services should balance local revenue-generating disparity, establish local capacity to provide minimum levels of service, and encourage local attention to state health objectives; support should include "core" funding. State funds could be furnished with strings attached and sanctions available for noncompliance, and/or general support could be provided with appropriate accountability requirements built in. States have the obligation in either case to monitor local use of state funds.

EDUCATION FOR PUBLIC HEALTH

Many educational paths can lead to careers in public health. However, the most direct educational path to a career in public health is to obtain a degree from a school of public health. Many of the 25 schools of public health are located in research universities and thus have a dual responsibility to develop knowledge and to produce well-trained professional practitioners. These dual roles are not always easy to balance.

Many observers feel that some schools have become somewhat isolated from public health practice and therefore no longer place a sufficiently high value on the training of professionals to work in health agencies. The dearth of professional agency leadership noted by the committee during the study may lend support to this view. The observed variations in agency practice, inadequate salaries, and frequently negative image of public health practice may partly account for any less-than-desirable responses by the educational institutions to the needs of practice.

In addition, most public health workers have no formal training in public health, and their need for basic grounding may not be appropriately met by the degree programs appropriate to prepare people for middle- and upper-level positions. To these ends the committee recommends:

- **Schools of public health should establish firm practice links with state and/or local public health agencies so that significantly more faculty members may undertake professional responsibilities in these agencies, conduct research there, and train students in such practice situations. Recruitment of faculty and admission of students should give appropriate weight to prior public health experience as well as to academic qualifications.**

- **Schools of public health should fulfill their potential role as significant resources to government at all levels in the development of public health policy.**

- **Schools of public health should provide students an opportunity to learn the entire scope of public health practice, including environmental, educational, and personal health approaches to the solution of public health problems; the basic epidemiological and biostatistical techniques for analysis of those problems; and the political and management skills needed for leadership in public health.**

- **Research in schools of public health should range from basic research in fields related to public health, through applied research and development, to program evaluation and implementation research.** The unique research mission of the schools of public health is to select research opportunities on the basis of their likely relevance to the solution of real public health problems and to test such applications in real life settings.

- **Schools of public health should take maximum advantage of training resources in their universities, for example, faculty and courses in schools of business administration, and departments of physical, biological, and social sciences.** The hazards of developing independent faculty resources isolated from the main disciplinary departments on the campus are real, and links between faculty in schools of public health and their parent disciplines should be sought and maintained.

- Because large numbers of persons being educated in other parts of the university will assume responsibilities in life that impact significantly on the public's health, e.g., involvement in production of hazardous goods or the enactment and enforcement of public health laws, **schools of public health** should extend their expertise to advise and assist with the health content of the educational programs of other schools and departments of the university.

• In view of the large numbers of personnel now engaged in public health without adequate preparation for their positions, **the schools of public health should undertake an expanded program of short courses to help upgrade the competence of these personnel.** In addition, short course offerings should provide opportunities for previously trained public health professionals, especially health officers, to keep up with advances in knowledge and practice.

• Because the schools of public health are not, and probably should not try to be, able to train the vast numbers of personnel needed for public health work, **the schools of public health should encourage and assist other institutions to prepare appropriate, qualified public health personnel for positions in the field.** When educational institutions other than schools of public health undertake to train personnel for work in the field, careful attention to the scope and capacity of the educational program is essential. This may be achieved in part by links with nearby schools of public health.

• **Schools of public health should strengthen their response to the needs for qualified personnel for important, but often neglected, aspects of public health such as the health of minority groups and international health.**

• **Schools of public health should help develop, or offer directly in their own universities, effective courses that expose undergraduates to concepts, history, current context, and techniques of public health to assist in the recruitment of able future leaders into the field.** The committee did not conclude whether undergraduate degrees in public health are useful.

• **Education programs for public health professionals should be informed by comprehensive and current data on public health personnel and their employment opportunities and needs.**

CONCLUDING REMARKS

This report conveys an urgent message to the American people. Public health is a vital function that is in trouble. Immediate public concern and support are called for in order to fulfill society's interest in assuring the conditions in which people can be healthy. History teaches us that an organized community effort to prevent disease and promote health is both valuable and effective. Yet public health in the United States has been taken for granted, many public health issues have become inappropriately politicized, and public health responsibilities have become so fragmented that deliberate action is often difficult if not impossible.

Restoring an effective public health system neither can nor should be achieved by public health professionals alone. Americans must be concerned that there are adequate public health services in their communities, and must let their elected representatives know of their concern. The specific actions appropriate to strengthen public health will vary from area to area and must blend professional knowledge with community values. The committee intends not to prescribe one best way of rescuing public health, but to admonish the readers to get involved in their own communities in order to address present dangers, now and for the sake of future generations.

1

The Disarray of Public Health: A Threat to the Health of the Public

This study was undertaken to address a growing perception among the Institute of Medicine membership and others concerned with the health of the public that this nation has lost sight of its public health goals and has allowed the system of public health activities to fall into disarray. Public health is what we, as a society, do collectively to assure the conditions for people to be healthy. This requires that continuing and emerging threats to the health of the public be successfully countered. These threats include immediate crises, such as the AIDS epidemic; enduring problems, such as injuries and chronic illness; and growing challenges, such as the aging of our population and the toxic by-products of a modern economy, transmitted through air, water, soil, or food.

These and many other problems raise in common the need to protect the nation's health through effective, organized, and sustained efforts led by the public sector. Unfortunately, the explorations of this committee, as documented in this report, confirm that our current capabilities for effective public health actions are inadequate. In the committee's view, we have let down our public health guard as a nation, and the health of the public is unnecessarily threatened as a result.

As a society we seem to assume that we are fully capable of maintaining past progress (often dramatic improvements in the public's health and longevity), of addressing current problems, and of being prepared to respond to new crises or emergent health problems. Instead, this committee has found a public health system that is incapable of meeting these responsibilities, of applying fully current scientific knowledge and organizational skills, and of generating new knowledge, methods, and programs.

The rest of this report sets out a conception of the vision that should guide the future of public health, analyzes the current situation and how it developed, and presents a plan of action that will, in the committee's judgment, provide a solid foundation for a strong public health capability throughout the nation. The strengthening of that capability requires understanding and support by many actors in this society, not just those in public health agencies. Therefore, the committee intends this report for a broad audience that includes elected public officials at all levels of government, voluntary health organizations, health care providers, educators of all of the health professions, and private citizens with interests in maintaining and improving health in their communities.

To help these broad audiences understand why we believe this topic is important to them and their communities, we begin by citing examples of specific threats that can be averted or lessened only through collective actions aimed at the community, in contrast with personal medical services initiated by patients or individual practitioners. These examples will serve to illustrate ultimate targets of public health activity. Improved organization, professional competence, and decisions about public interventions are valued not as ends in themselves, but as means to combat real dangers to the public's health.

IMMEDIATE CRISES

The following are examples of problems that constitute immediate crises and can only be solved by collective action. Both examples are major current concerns for most public health agencies throughout the nation.

AIDS (ACQUIRED IMMUNE DEFICIENCY SYNDROME)

The infectious disease of AIDS, caused by the human immunodeficiency virus (HIV), became an epidemic in little more than 5 years after its discovery. The virus now infects more than a million people in the United States and millions more in other countries. The cases of AIDS reported thus far are only the beginning of the expected toll because of the long period between infection and overt disease. A sizable proportion of those now infected will progress to severe disease and death. (Figure 1.1; Committee on a National Strategy for AIDS, Institute of Medicine, and National Academy of Sciences, 1986)

As noted by the Institute of Medicine and National Academy of Sciences in their 1986 report, the unchecked spread of HIV could convert the current epidemic into a catastrophe. To slow the spread until a vaccine or definitive treatment is developed, the report recommended that the United States

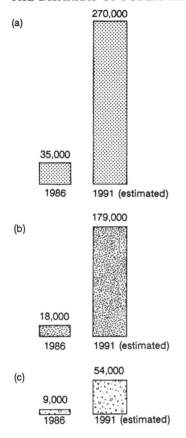

FIGURE 1.1 (a) Cumulative cases of AIDS in the United States at the end of the year. (b) Cumulative deaths in the United States at the end of the year. (c) Deaths in the United States during the year. SOURCE: Committee on a National Strategy for AIDS, Institute of Medicine, and National Academy of Sciences, 1986, Appendix G, p. 328.

undertake a massive media, educational, and public health campaign. This campaign would include effective education to inform the public of the danger and to describe changes in behavior that can minimize the risk of infection, voluntary testing to identify persons infected with the virus, and counseling of infected persons in order to contain the spread. (Committee on a National Strategy for AIDS, Institute of Medicine, and National Academy of Sciences, 1986) More than any other event of recent years, the AIDS epidemic has reminded us of the necessity of effective public health actions to protect individuals and society.

ACCESS TO HEALTH CARE FOR THE INDIGENT

About 43 million Americans, or 18 percent of the population, do not have a physician, clinic, or hospital as a regular source of health care. Some 38.8 million Americans, or 16 percent of the population, have difficulty obtaining health care when they need it. Half these people have difficulty because they are unable to pay for care. (The Robert Wood Johnson Foundation, 1987)

Those who cannot afford health care—the medically indigent—include poor and near poor, employed and unemployed, uninsured and underinsured. They include children, adults, and the elderly. A survey in 1986 conducted by The Robert Wood Johnson Foundation estimated that some 22 million Americans did not have health insurance, public or private. (The Robert Wood Johnson Foundation, 1987) About half of these people are employed but not insured; the other half are unemployed. (The Robert Wood Johnson Foundation, 1985) Of those citizens with incomes below the federal poverty line, fewer than half receive Medicaid. Those who do receive Medicaid may be covered only for selected services. In many states, Medicaid covers basic hospital and ambulatory services, but not other basic needs such as dental services. (Desonia and King, 1985) The proportion of persons below the poverty line who do not receive Medicaid increased from 47 percent in 1975 to about 54 percent in 1985. (The Robert Wood Johnson Foundation, 1985) The proportion of persons with no regular source of health care has increased substantially, by 65 percent, in the past 5 years. And the proportion of citizens who had health problems but refrained from making an ambulatory visit in the course of a year increased by 70 percent in the past 5 years. (The Robert Wood Johnson Foundation, 1987)

The 1986 survey documented the difficulties that poor Americans encounter in obtaining health care. Despite their generally worse health status, the indigent are less likely to have a regular source of health care, are less likely to be insured, and are less likely to receive health care services than more affluent persons. The better-off population made 37 percent more ambulatory visits to health care facilities than did poor persons of similar health status. Yet it has been well documented that the indigent tend to have more illnesses and disabilities than more affluent citizens. It has also been documented that the gap between rich and poor is widening.

Access to health care services in this country has become a crisis both for the population that has difficulty obtaining care and for providers of care, the latter often publicly owned or financed, and the growing reluctance of private health care institutions to provide free care is placing an increasing financial burden on public institutions. The evidence shows that many Americans are going without needed health care. Since 1984, more than half the states have passed legislation concerned with the health care needs of the medically indigent. More than 20 states have appointed commissions to study means of providing care. (Desonia and King, 1985) This issue promises to be a critical problem throughout the 1980s.

When the uninsured and poor do seek health care, the burden of providing this care falls disproportionately on a small number of institutions, often the public providers of health care. Ten percent of the hospitals in the country provide more than 40 percent of all inpatient and ambulatory health care services to the uninsured. (The Robert Wood Johnson Foundation, 1985) Studies in several cities indicate that an overwhelming proportion of the medically indigent are admitted or transferred to public hospitals and university hospitals when seeking care. These hospitals, in turn, are in increasing financial jeopardy. (Annas, 1986) The burden of ambulatory care for the uninsured and poor is also carried by community clinics and public health departments. For a subset of these people, the problems are compounded by homelessness (IOM study, to be published).

ENDURING PUBLIC HEALTH PROBLEMS

Although such immediate crises as AIDS and care of the indigent tend to attract attention of the public and of policymakers, other public health problems with equally great significance for the health of the public and the well-being of our society require continuing attention. Progress against an enduring problem may lead to complacency, and the very permanency of the problem may undermine continued vigilance and actions. The four examples given here have all been targets of concerted action through public efforts, and some progress has been achieved. Yet maintenance of that progress and continued advances require sustained effort.

INJURIES

William Foege, former director of the federal Centers for Disease Control, has stated that injury is the principal public health problem in America today, affecting primarily the young, and will touch one of every three Americans each year.

Each year, more than 140,000 Americans die from injuries and another 70 million sustain nonfatal injuries. Injury is the leading cause of death for children and young adults. Motor vehicle accidents are the leading cause of severe injury and death, causing about 3.2 million injuries in 1982 and about one-third of the fatal deaths each year. (Figure 1.2; Committee on Trauma Research, Commission on Life Sciences, National Research Council, and Institute of Medicine, 1985)

We have not done enough to reduce this toll. Public action can reduce injuries by:

—education that persuades people to protect themselves from injury;

—legal requirements for desirable protective actions, such as auto seat belt use or the use of smoke detectors; and

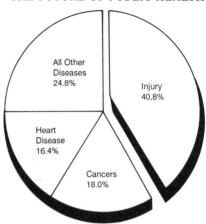

FIGURE 1.2 Percentages of years of potential life lost to injury, cancer, heart disease, and other diseases before age 65. Modified from Centers for Disease Control. SOURCE: Committee on Trauma Research, Commission on Life Sciences, National Research Council, and Institute of Medicine, *Injury in America: A Continuing Public Health Problem,* 1985, p. 20.

—protection through product and environmental design, e.g., highway safety standards, automatic seat belts or air bags, sprinkler systems, child-proof caps on medicines, and so on. (Committee on Trauma Research, Commission on Life Sciences, National Research Council, and Institute of Medicine, 1985)

TEEN PREGNANCY

About half a million babies are born each year to teenage mothers in the United States. Births to teenagers represented about 13 percent of all births in the nation in 1984. Rates of teen pregnancy and delivery in the United States are significantly higher than those of comparable countries. For example, 15-year-old girls in the United States are 5 times more likely to get pregnant than girls in any other developed country for which data are available. (Panel on Adolescent Pregnancy and Childbearing, Committee on Child Development, Research and Public Policy, Commission on Behavioral and Social Sciences and Education, National Research Council, 1987)

The number of births to teenage mothers in this country has serious public health implications. Pregnant teenagers have higher rates of miscarriages, complications, stillbirths, and infant and maternal deaths than pregnant adults. Low-income teenagers are more likely than adults to have premature births, increasing the likelihood of poor pregnancy outcomes. (Committee to Study the Prevention of Low Birthweight, Institute of Medicine, 1985) Surviving children of teenage mothers are more likely to suffer injuries and more likely to be hospitalized by age 5 than children of adult mothers. Adolescent pregnancies and births cause significant health problems both for teenage mothers and for their children. In addition, teenage pregnancy is linked to school dropout, contributing to low future incomes, which are in turn associated with poorer health in future years. (Panel on Adolescent Pregnancy and Childbearing, Committee on Child Development, Research and Public Policy, Commission on Behavioral and Social Sciences and Education, National Research Council, 1987)

Many of the health problems associated with early pregnancy and childbearing can be significantly reduced with proper prenatal care and nutrition. Yet adolescents are the least likely mothers to receive prenatal care. (Panel on Adolescent Pregnancy and Childbearing, Committee on Child Development, Research and Public Policy, Commission on Behavioral and Social Sciences and Education, National Research Council, 1987) Only about half of all teen mothers begin prenatal care in their first trimester of pregnancy, and about 12 percent never receive any prenatal care. (Hughes et al., 1986) Also, teenagers are far more likely to have poor eating habits. Moreover, most teenage parents have difficulty in financing health care for themselves and for their children. In many locations, teenage girls rely on public health agencies for health services. Family planning services offered by many public health agencies as well as by private providers can prevent unwanted pregnancies but are underutilized. When pregnancies do occur, efforts in health education and maternal and child health services are needed to improve pregnancy outcomes. (Panel on Adolescent Pregnancy and Childbearing, Committee on Child Development, Research and Public Policy, Commission on Behavioral and Social Sciences and Education, National Research Council, 1987)

CONTROL OF HIGH BLOOD PRESSURE

Public health measures, once associated mainly with control of infectious disease, can also be effective against chronic diseases. Epidemiological and statistical studies have established factors associated with high risk from heart disease and stroke. One of these risk factors is high blood pressure, which affects about 60 million Americans. (Office of Disease Prevention and Health Promotion, Office of the Assistant Secretary for Health, Public Health Service, U.S. Department of Health and Human Services, 1983) In 1972, the Public Health Service mounted a national campaign to identify the population afflicted with high blood pressure and to lower the blood pressure levels. (Roccella, 1985) The success of that campaign, which involved private agencies as well as national, state, and local public health agencies, is illustrated by the increased control of high blood pressure (see Figure 1.3). The progress in reducing high blood pressure has undoubtedly contributed to the considerable reduction in the incidence of stroke between 1972 and 1982 (see Figure 1.4).

(a)

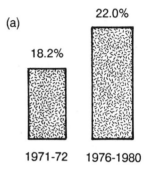

22.0%

18.2%

1971-72   1976-1980

(b)

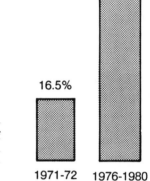

34.1%

16.5%

FIGURE 1.3   (a) Prevalence of high blood pressure for persons 25–74 years of age in the United States. (b) Proportion of persons with high blood pressure whose disease is controlled (aware and adequately treated). SOURCE: Lenfant and Roccella, 1984, p. 460.

1971-72   1976-1980

Continued public health efforts will be required to maintain this progress because the incidence of uncontrolled hypertension is still very substantial. Up to two-thirds of those with hypertension in 1976–1980 were not in control programs. (Lenfant and Roccella, 1984) In 1986, high blood pressure control rates varied among communities from 25 to 60 percent. (Office of Disease Prevention and Health Promotion, Public Health Service, U.S. Department of Health and Human Services, 1986)

SMOKING AND SUBSTANCE ABUSE

Thirty percent of American adults are addicted to cigarettes. Cigarette smokers have a 70 percent higher death rate from all causes than non-smokers. Smoking is the single greatest cause of premature death in this country. It is estimated that smoking contributes to as many as 225,000 deaths from coronary heart disease, 100,000 deaths from cancers, and 20,000 deaths from chronic obstructive lung disease each year. Additionally,

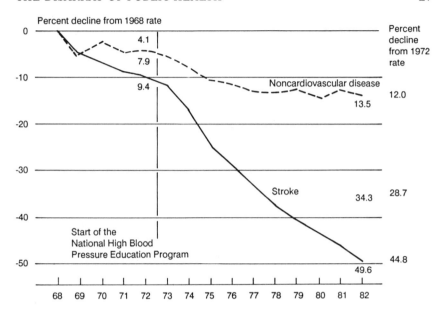

FIGURE 1.4   Death from stroke. SOURCE: Roccella, 1985, p. 655.

10 million Americans suffer from debilitating chronic diseases caused by smoking. (Office of Disease Prevention and Health Promotion, Office of the Assistant Secretary for Health, Public Health Service, U.S. Department of Health and Human Services, 1983) Also, smoking is the major identifiable cause of residential fire deaths and injuries in the country and is associated with higher injury and chemical illness risk in many occupations. About 30 percent of all adults and about 20 percent of high schoolers in the United States regularly smoke cigarettes, but those proportions have decreased from 33 percent of adults and 27 percent of high school teenagers in 1979. (Office of Disease Prevention and Health Promotion, Office of the Assistant Secretary for Health, Public Health Service, U.S. Department of Health and Human Services, 1986)

Annual per capita alcohol consumption in the United States has remained steady, at slightly under 3 gallons per person age 14 and over since 1978. But alcoholism may be on the rise. For example, 1982 data indicate that as many as 41 percent of teenagers engage in occasional binge drinking, an increase from 37 percent in 1975. (Office of Disease Prevention and Health Promotion, Office of the Assistant Secretary for Health, Public Health Service, U.S. Department of Health and Human Services, 1986)

During the late 1970s and early 1980s, drug use remained relatively stable and even declined for some substances. About 16 million Americans regularly smoke marijuana, 1 to 2 million regularly use cocaine, 1 million misuse barbiturates, and thousands are addicted to heroin. (Office of Disease Prevention and Health Promotion, Office of the Assistant Secretary for Health, Public Health Service, U.S. Department of Health and Human Services, 1983) Between 1977 and 1982, use of marijuana in young adults declined from about 19 percent to about 16 percent, and from 9 percent to 6 percent in teenagers. But use of other drugs by adults, particularly cocaine, more than doubled, from under 1 percent to over 2 percent. (Office of Disease Prevention and Health Promotion, Office of the Assistant Secretary for Health, Public Health Service, U.S. Department of Health and Human Services, 1983)

Alcohol and drug abuse are major factors in much illness, disability, and death in the United States. Some problems are immediate, and some evolve over a period of time. Ten percent of all deaths in the United States are related to alcohol use. Cirrhosis of the liver, which is largely attributable to alcohol use, caused 10.7 deaths per 100,000 population in 1984. Alcohol abuse is also frequently related to motor vehicle injuries and deaths. In 1984, the death rate from alcohol-related motor vehicle accidents was 9.5 per 100,000, and from other alcohol-related accidents, 4.3 per 100,000. Drug abuse has also been related to premature death, severe physical disability, psychological disability, homicides, suicides, and injuries. In 1984, it was estimated that there were more than 3,500 drug-related deaths in 26 major metropolitan areas of the United States. Drug use causes some 100,000 to 350,000 hospital admissions per year. (Office of Disease Prevention and Health Promotion, Office of the Assistant Secretary for Health, Public Health Service, U.S. Department of Health and Human Services, 1986) Intravenous drug use also is a major risk factor for contracting AIDS virus infection from contaminated needles and syringes. The three habits of smoking, alcohol abuse, and drug abuse have consistently been related to poor pregnancy outcomes.

Despite some declining trends in substance abuse, the health effects of current and previous use will be felt for years to come. There is some indication that public health measures directed toward controlling substance abuse, including health education of the public and of health professionals, have contributed to the reductions in substance abuse mentioned above. In general, in the early 1980s more adults and teenagers reported awareness of the dangers of smoking, alcohol abuse, and drug abuse than had in the late 1970s. But an ongoing effort will be required to reduce the long-term burden on the public health caused by substance abuse.

GROWING CHALLENGES AND IMPENDING CRISES

Some health problems are likely to be increased by factors that are already identifiable. These "time bombs" of public health include the following two examples.

TOXIC SUBSTANCES

The problem of hazardous waste generated by industry becomes bigger with each new discovery of environmental contamination from improper disposal of toxic materials. Contamination exists in ground water, air, soil, and food and has serious implications for public health. (Walker, 1985)

Most toxic substances are present in more than one medium and may be readily transferred from air to soil to food and water. For example, when residues from waste water treatment plants are incinerated, a portion of the pollutants is converted to air pollutants, which in turn contaminate water and soil.

Pollution of groundwater and other drinking water supplies is a serious threat to public health. For example, for nearly 17 years, until voluntary closure in 1972, the Stringfellow acid pit near Riverside, California, accepted about 35 million gallons of industrial waste. Thirteen years after the site stopped receiving toxic waste and 5 years after the pits were capped, a major groundwater basin was still being contaminated. Various containment efforts were made to prevent these wastes from migrating. These old technologies failed at this site as they have at other waste holding pits. (Embers, 1985)

Pesticides contaminate many common American foods (tomatoes, beef, potatoes, oranges, lettuce) and may be responsible for some cancers, according to *Regulating Pesticides in Foods: The Delaney Paradox,* a National Academy of Sciences report released in 1987. That study focused on 28 of the 53 pesticides classified as carcinogenic or potentially carcinogenic. More than 80 percent of those analyzed exceeded the Environmental Protection Agency threshold of acceptable cancer risk for an environmental toxicant—no more than one additional case of cancer for every 1 million persons exposed. (Board on Agriculture, National Academy of Sciences, 1987)

Although recent attention has been focused mainly on cancer, the range of adverse human health effects of exposure to chemicals and other toxic substances is broad. Exposure to high levels of some substances for even short periods may produce acute, though often temporary, effects such as rash, burns, or poisoning. Prolonged exposure to low doses can cause lung disease and neurobehavioral disorders. There is growing evidence that environmental toxicants can cause reproductive problems, including miscarriages and birth defects. An increased incidence of abortion and stillbirth among women exposed to high lead concentrations has long been recognized. Studies of mercury and aluminum indicate that these metals, too, may affect pregnancy outcome. The National Institute of Occupational Safety and Health reports that more than 4 million workers are directly exposed to those metals that can cause chronic kidney disease. (Walker, 1985; National Academy of Engineering, 1986)

Controlling toxic substances in the environment will continue to present new challenges for the legal and the public health systems of the nation. With growing evidence of the human health effects of some toxic substances, the number of lawsuits and other efforts to obtain compensation by injured parties will rise. Implementation of federal toxic substances control laws, such as the Toxic Substance Control Act (TSCA) and the Federal Insecticide, Fungicide and Rodenticide Act, has raised numerous questions concerning testing of thousands of chemicals in commercial use, including who should test them, when they should be tested, and for what effects they should be tested. These and similar issues have slowed the rate at which the laws can be implemented. (Embers, 1985; Walker, 1985)

ALZHEIMER'S DISEASE OR DEMENTIA OF THE ALZHEIMER TYPE

As many as 2 million Americans are suffering from Alzheimer's disease, resulting in severe, disabling intellectual impairment. The exact causes of Alzheimer's are unknown, but it is clearly associated with age. (Katzman, 1986) Although a small percentage of those under age 60 are believed to have Alzheimer's, more than 20 percent of the population over age 80 is believed to have the disease. The prevalence of cases of Alzheimer's increases 10- to 20-fold between age 60 and age 80 years. (Secretary's Task Force on Alzheimer's Disease, U.S. Department of Health and Human Services, 1984)

The number of Alzheimer's disease cases is expected to increase dramatically over the next several decades as the population ages. The elderly are the most rapidly growing group within our population, and, within that group, the proportion of elderly age 85 and over is increasing the most rapidly. In 1980, the elderly population in the United States (age 65 and over) numbered some 26 million, or about 11 percent of the population. By the year 2025, as the baby boom of the mid-twentieth century reaches old age, the elderly population is expected to reach a peak of 58.5 million people, or a full 20 percent of the population. (Secretary's Task Force on Alzheimer's Disease, U.S. Department of Health and Human Services, 1984)

The association between Alzheimer's dementia and the aging of the population will increase greatly the demand for long-term care. Currently, over half of the million and a half residents of nursing homes are estimated to have Alzheimer's disease. (Katzman, 1986) Many others are cared for in sheltered housing or day care facilities. When care is provided by family members or friends, the care givers themselves may suffer economic deprivation or declines in physical or mental health status. Although considerable research is being done on the causes of Alzheimer's, it is likely that treatment of the disease will continue to require some form of long-term health care. (Katzman, 1986) Alzheimer's represents a particular challenge to public health leadership to assure access to and quality of appropriate services.

REVITALIZATION OF PUBLIC HEALTH CAPACITIES

To counter these and other threats to the health of the public will require a vital and effective public health system capable of the full range of responses necessary to make further progress against disease, disability, and premature death. Controlling communicable disease, encouraging healthy lifestyles, reducing hazards in the environment, and targeting and assuring necessary personal health and long-term care services—all of the classic tools of public health—are necessary to maintain the benefits of past success and to respond to current and future challenges.

The successes of past public health efforts are many. The virtual elimination of many infectious diseases, such as typhoid fever and paralytic polio; great reductions in many of the common childhood communicable diseases (Committee on Public-Private Sector Relations in Vaccine Innovation, Institute of Medicine, 1985); and initial progress in the control of common chronic diseases, such as heart disease, stroke, and some forms of cancer (Office of Disease Prevention and Health Promotion, Public Health Service, U.S. Department of Health and Human Services, 1986), are ample evidence of the effectiveness of public health measures that join scientific knowledge and effective social action. However, the success of past efforts can lead to complacency about the need for a vigorous public health enterprise at the national, state, and local levels. **To achieve public health objectives, public health will need to serve as leader and catalyst of private efforts as well as performing those health functions that only government can perform.** The committee believes firmly that the substantial improvements in health status that are the result of public health activities require vigorous, scientifically competent, politically astute, comprehensive, and sustained public health capacity.

It is, therefore, with great concern and some alarm that the committee has observed the current state of public health. We have observed many symptoms of systemic problems, solutions to which will require a comprehensive strategy and a strong commitment on the part of the entire society. We have observed disorganization, weak and unstable leadership, a lessening of professional and expert competence in leadership positions, hostility to public health concepts and approaches, outdated statutes, inadequate financial support for public health activities and public health education, gaps in the data gathering and analysis that are essential to the public health functions of assessment and surveillance, and lack of effective links between the public and private sectors for the accomplishment of public health objectives.

In our view, these problems reflect a lack of appreciation among the general public and policymakers for the crucial role that a strong public health capacity must play in maintaining and improving the health of the public. Attention is focused on specific health problems such as AIDS, exposure to specific toxic agents, or substance abuse. But these specific foci of interest lead to episodic actions, not to the sustained effort that is needed. The necessary public health capacity to cope with the immediate, enduring, and impending threats to health cannot, in the committee's view, be turned on and off as particular health problems arise and receive attention. This necessary capacity must be nurtured and supported by the society that reaps the benefits; it requires competent people, effective leadership, a scientifically sound knowledge base, the tools to monitor health problems and measure progress, a productive organizational structure, adequate financial resources, and a legal foundation that supports effective action, all motivated by a vision of the public's health that is understood and supported by that public. By its very nature, public health requires support by members of the public—its beneficiaries. While individual action to improve health is necessary, it is not enough, and, as the above examples illustrate, health status will fall short of the achievable if public health is not strong.

To provide a comprehensive and well-founded strategy to overcome the current disarray, the rest of this volume will examine and reaffirm the concepts of public health, develop a desirable framework for public health action, assess the current status of public health as an organized activity in the United States, and finally, recommend specific actions and directions that will provide a vigorous and effective public health enterprise sufficient to the challenges that lie ahead.

REFERENCES

Annas, George J. 1986. "Your Money or Your Life: 'Dumping' Uninsured Patients from Hospital Emergency Wards." *American Journal of Public Health* 76(1):74–77.

Board on Agriculture, National Academy of Sciences. 1987. *Regulating Pesticides in Foods: The Delaney Paradox.* National Academy Press, Washington, D.C.

Committee on a National Strategy for AIDS, Institute of Medicine, and National Academy of Sciences. 1986. *Confronting AIDS: Directions for Public Health, Health Care, and Research.* National Academy Press, Washington, D.C.

Committee on Public-Private Sector Relations in Vaccine Innovation, Institute of Medicine, 1985. *Vaccine Supply and Innovation,* National Academy Press, Washington, D.C.

Committee on Trauma Research, Commission on Life Sciences, National Research Council, and Institute of Medicine. 1985. *Injury in America: A Continuing Public Health Problem.* National Academy Press, Washington, D.C.

Committee to Study the Prevention of Low Birthweight, Institute of Medicine. 1985. *Preventing Low Birthweight.* National Academy Press, Washington, D.C.

Desonia, Randolph A., and Kathleen M. King. 1985. *State Programs of Assistance for the Medically Indigent.* Intergovernmental Health Policy Project, Washington, D.C.

Embers, L. R. 1985. "Clean-up Mishaps Show Need to Alter Superfund Law." *Chemical and Engineering News* 63(21):11–21, May 27.

Hughes, Dana, Kay Johnson, Janet Simons, and Sara Rosenbaum. 1986. *Maternal and Child Health Data Book: The Health of American's Children.* Children's Defense Fund, Washington, D.C.

Katzman, Robert. 1986. "Alzheimer's Disease." *New England Journal of Medicine* 314(15):964–973.

Lenfant, Claude, and Edward Roccella. 1984. "Trends in Hypertension Control in the United States." *Chest* 86:459–462, September.

National Academy of Engineering. 1986. *Hazards: Technology and Fairness.* National Academy Press, Washington, D.C.

Office of Disease Prevention and Health Promotion, Office of the Assistant Secretary for Health, Public Health Service, U.S. Department of Health and Human Services. 1983. *Public Health Service Implementation Plans for Obtaining Objectives for the Nation.* Public Health Reports, supplement to the September–October 1983 Issue.

Office of Disease Prevention and Health Promotion, Public Health Service, U.S. Department of Health and Human Services. 1986. *The 1990 Objectives for the Nation: A Midcourse Review.* U.S. Department of Health and Human Services, Washington, D.C.

Panel on Adolescent Pregnancy and Childbearing, Committee on Child Development, Research and Public Policy, Commission on Behavioral and Social Sciences Education, National Research Council. 1987. *Risking the Future: Adolescent Sexuality, Pregnancy, and Childbearing,* Cheryl D. Hayes, ed. National Academy Press, Washington, D.C.

The Robert Wood Johnson Foundation. 1985. *Announcing the Health Care for the Uninsured Program.* Brochure. The Robert Wood Johnson Foundation.

The Robert Wood Johnson Foundation. 1987. *Access to Health Care in the United States: Results of a 1986 Survey.* Special Report Number 2. The Robert Wood Johnson Foundation.

Roccella, Edward J. 1985. "Meeting the 1990 Hypertension Objectives for the Nation: A Progress Report." *Public Health Reports* 100(6):652–56, November–December.

Secretary's Task Force on Alzheimer's Disease, U.S. Department of Health and Human Services. 1984. *Alzheimer's Disease.* U.S. Government Printing Office, Washington, D.C.

Walker, B. 1985. "The Present Role of the Local Health Department in Environmental Toxicology." *Journal of Environmental Health* 48(3):133–137, November–December.

2

A Vision of Public Health in America: An Attainable Ideal

The discussion in Chapter 1 implicitly asked, "Why be concerned about public health?" and gave two broad answers.

The first answer focused on present threats to the health of the public. Urgent new problems like AIDS and toxic wastes have been added to the public health agenda. At the same time, a changing U.S. health system has brought more sharply into focus the unsolved dilemma of how to care for some 30 million uninsured and underinsured Americans, and has called into question old understandings about the respective roles of the private and public sectors. These new concerns have heightened competition for scarce financial resources and public attention and support. Americans assume that government is equipped to fulfill its obligation to protect the public from such threats. But the nation's public health capacity has become seriously weakened, and public support—always fragile because of limited awareness—is increasingly being eroded by controversy.

The second answer pointed to past achievements as the basis for believing that public health still retains fundamental problem-solving capacity. Historically, public health has made a difference in the quality of life for all Americans. Governmental actions to assure the health of the people—such as water quality control, immunizations, and food inspection—have prevented much illness and many deaths. These traditional and ongoing accomplishments have demonstrated the value of public health efforts, and exemplify the kind of success that is possible as a result of organized effort on the basis of technical knowledge. If they demonstrate the best of which public health has been capable, they also underscore the urgency of rescuing this vital public capacity from its current decline.

Chapters 3 and 4 give a more detailed picture of the current status of U.S. public health. They spell out its history, organization, current activities, and problems. But first, the observation that something is *wrong* with public health implies some sense of what would be *right:* a vision against which to assess current realities and guide decisions about what changes should be made. "Vision" as used here is not meant to suggest a form of impractical utopianism that results in a set of impossible dreams. Instead, the aim is to fashion in the mind's eye—as the prerequisite to doing so in reality—an attainable ideal.

This chapter sets forth the committee's vision of public health. It presents the value framework in which it has reflected about the present dilemma of public health and formed its recommendations. The vision appears early in the report to encourage readers to weigh this ideal while they reflect on public health as described in the report and as they view it in their own communities. The committee hopes readers will ask themselves not only whether or not they share the values or agree with the conclusions in this report, but also how closely the current reality of public health approximates their own ideal model and what they can do to move practice in directions they consider sound.

The committee's vision of public health includes the following conceptual elements:

A definition of "public health" that the committee believes is consistent with key American values. This definition sets forth the committee's view of what the term "public health" should mean and what values are implied by that understanding. The definition has three parts:

1. The mission of public health: a statement of ultimate goals or purposes. This section addresses the question: What are the common goals of public health?

2. The substance of public health: a statement about subject matter. This section addresses the question: What areas of concern does public health deal with?

3. The organizational framework of public health: a statement that distinguishes the concerns included in the term "public health" from the ways in which society organizes to deal with them. This section addresses the question: How is "public health" different from "what public health agencies do?"

The governmental functions of public health. Federal, state, and local agencies as institutions of government have unique authority, obligations, and duties. This section discusses public health as a government responsibility. It considers:

1. the duties that are essential to government's responsibility for public health;

2. the expression of these duties at the federal, state, and local levels; and

3. the relationship between government and the private sector.

The basic services of public health. This section discusses the activities, tasks, programs, and benefits that are required to address the mission of public health. In contrast to functions that are specific to the role of the public agency, responsibility for the provision of basic services is shared by public and private sectors.

Figure 2.1 is a diagram of how the conceptual elements of the public health vision relate to one another.

A DEFINITION OF PUBLIC HEALTH

"When I think of public health, I think of early intervention, prevention."

"Public health is immunization, school health, control of contagious disease."

"It's anything that affects the health of the community on a mass basis."

"Public health is the area of health outside the capability of the individual private practitioner."

"The core of public health is the capacity to identify problems, and having found them, measure them and attempt to intervene."*

The quotations above, gathered during the course of this study, illustrate that the effort to define public health is complex. When asked, people tend to mix observations about what actual health departments do with assertions about what society as a whole ought to do. Some emphasize a community focus, in contrast to individual patient care. Others concentrate on ideas of government response to market failure. Still others list the contents of practice, such as control of environmental hazards or care of the poor, or refer to professional skills, such as epidemiology or sanitary engineering.

As we will see in Chapters 3 and 4, this variety of definitions is exceeded— and perhaps also explained—by the complexity of the system in which, somewhere, "public health" is found. The United States is notable among the countries of the world for complicated policy relationships among national, state, and local levels of government and for its interweaving of private and public sector activity. Health affairs share in this complexity. Given this intricate arrangement, the committee hopes that a clear definition will help those who work in, are served by, or study the system to sort out its elements, understand it, and work to make it perform more effectively.

From the beginning of its work, the committee believed that it was important not to limit understanding of "public health" to what health depart-

---

* These and following quotations are taken from interviews conducted during the course of the study. See Chapter 4 for a description of study activities.

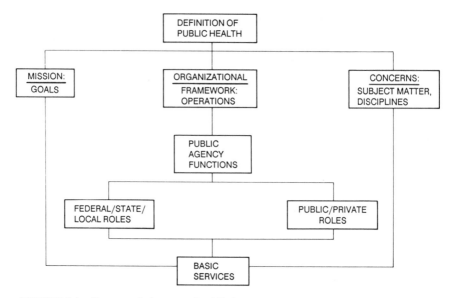

FIGURE 2.1 Conceptual elements of public health.

ments do. Instead, it aimed to place government activities within a broader framework that can guide a wide range of institutional participants. The intent is not to deemphasize the role of the public agency. On the contrary, it is to point out the indispensability of its prerogatives and functions by calling attention to the context in which they are exercised. This distinction between "public health" and "what health departments do" is reinforced by dividing the definition into three parts. By separating the *organizational expression* of public health from understandings of its *mission* and *subject matter,* the committee intends to emphasize that the goals and concerns of public health can and should be addressed not only by health departments, but also by private organizations and practitioners, other public agencies, and the community at large. The governing role of the official public health agency in assuring that the overall system works is, however, indispensable.

THE MISSION OF PUBLIC HEALTH

In eighteenth- and early nineteenth-century America, public health measures were taken in response to particular epidemic crises. Thus the earliest definition of public health's mission was practical rather than formal: control of epidemic disease. The first explicit statement came with the justly famous Shattuck Report of 1850, which declared "the conditions of perfect health, either public or personal" to be the goal of public health. (Rosenkrantz, 1972)

One of the earliest deliberate efforts to define public health's mission is still one of the most frequently cited. According to C. E. A. Winslow (as quoted in Hanlon and Pickett, 1984):

Public health is the science and the art of (1) preventing disease, (2) prolonging life, and (3) organized community efforts for (a) the sanitation of the environment, (b) the control of communicable infections, (c) the education of the individual in personal hygiene, (d) the organization of medical and nursing services for the early diagnosis and preventive treatment of disease, and (e) the development of the social machinery to ensure everyone a standard of living adequate for the maintenance of health, so organizing these benefits as to enable every citizen to realize his birthright of health and longevity.

More recently, Ellencweig and Yoshpe have conceived the goal of public health to be protection of the community against the hazards engendered by group life. (Ellencweig and Yoshpe, 1984) Beauchamp sees the mission of public health as social justice and the protection of all human life. (Beauchamp, 1976)

The common themes that run through these interpretations are reflected in the words "public" and "health." What unites people around public health is the focus on society as a whole, the community, and the aim of optimal health status.

Clearly, public health is "public" because it involves "organized community effort." It is not simply the outcome of isolated individual efforts. Its mission is to ensure that organized approaches are mobilized when they are needed. For example, both smallpox vaccination of countless individuals and treatment of unvaccinated patients would not have rid us of smallpox without strategies aimed specifically at the communitywide (in this case, the worldwide) level, such as epidemiologic studies, consistent reporting of cases, and organized distribution of vaccine. In a similar way, neither treatment of lung disease nor exhorting individuals to avoid smoking could have achieved the reduction of smoking in public places made possible by organized community effort to adopt laws and regulations restricting smoking. Seat belt legislation is still another instance in which a communitywide approach has augmented individual effort.

Public health is also public in terms of its long-range goal, which is optimal health for the entire community. This goal encompasses both the sum of the health status of individual community members and communitywide benefits such as clean air and water. The "health" aspect of the public health mission is perhaps best understood by reference to the well-known World Health Organization (WHO) definition. WHO has defined health as "a state of complete well-being, physical, social, and mental, and not merely the absence of disease or infirmity." (World Health Organization, as quoted by Hanlon and Pickett, 1984) Our shared sense of what "complete well-being" might be, though none of us has ever experienced it, serves as a focus for commitment to extend community efforts beyond the narrow concerns of special interests and the boundaries of any one professional discipline.

The committee's own definition takes into consideration all of the dimensions outlined above. The committee defines the *mission* of public health as: the fulfillment of society's interest in assuring the conditions in which people can be healthy.

THE SUBSTANCE OF PUBLIC HEALTH

Within this mission fall a number of characteristic themes, which over the course of a long historical tradition have coalesced around the goal of the people's health. Early public health focused on sanitary measures and the control of communicable disease. With the discovery of bacteria and immunologic advances, disease prevention was added to the subject matter of public health. (Hanlon and Pickett, 1984) In recent decades, health promotion has become an increasingly important theme, as the interrelationship among the physical, mental, and social dimensions of well-being has been clarified. Over time, the substance of public health has expanded. A 1985 editorial in the *Journal of Public Health Policy* pointed out that a commitment to multidimensional well-being implies the need to address factors that fall outside the normal understanding of "health," including decent housing, public education, adequate income, freedom from war, and so on. (Terris, 1986) While encouraging a holistic approach, this tendency to widen the boundaries of public health has the effect of forcing practitioners to make difficult choices about where to focus their energies and raises the possibility that public health could be so broadly defined so as to lose distinctive meaning.

Even restricting public health's subject matter to disease prevention and control, health promotion, and environmental measures necessitates the involvement of a broad spectrum of professional disciplines. In fact, it is frequently pointed out that public health is a coalition of professions united by their shared mission (described in the section above); their focus on disease prevention and health promotion; their prospective approach in contrast to the reactive focus of therapeutic medicine (Draper et al., as quoted in Hanlon and Pickett, 1984); and their common science, epidemiology:

Each [profession] brings to the public health task the distinctive skills of a primary professional discipline; but, in addition, each shares a distinctive and unique body of knowledge . . .

The mother science of public health is epidemiology, i.e., the systematic, objective study of the natural history of disease within populations and the factors that determine its spread. (as quoted by Terris, 1985)

Epidemiology is the "glue" that holds public health's many professions together. It is by means of the application of scientific and technical knowledge, above all else, that public health practitioners strive to improve the lot of humankind, to understand the causes of disease, to identify populations at risk, and to develop new approaches to prevention. (Robbins, 1985)

Thus the committee defines the *substance* of public health as: organized community efforts aimed at the prevention of disease and promotion of health. It links many disciplines and rests upon the scientific core of epidemiology.

THE ORGANIZATIONAL FRAMEWORK OF PUBLIC HEALTH

Specific attention to the organizational framework for public health activities is important because many Americans support the goals of public health but are highly critical of a particular health department.

During the course of the study, when committee members and staff told people that its subject was "the future of public health," the most common first question they received was, "Do you mean what health departments do, or are you talking about public health in general?" For many people the normal range of health department activities, whatever the level of government under study, does not adequately define "public health." Clearly, the committee sees public health as more than what health departments do and perceives important roles for the private sector and for public-private partnerships in the future of public health, as subsequent discussion will amplify. But the tone of some site visit conversations (see Chapters 3 and 4) suggests another consideration. Numerous comments implied not only that the *content* of public health's future might vary depending on whether the reference point is health departments or a broader set of entities, but its likely *quality*—the prognosis—might also be different. In other words, as site visits have illustrated, while the mission and substance of public health appear to have wide support around the country, the health department frequently does not. There appears to be a gap between popular support for public health concerns and public confidence in the value and effectiveness of current health department activities. People tend to be positive about public health values, but negative about the present public health agency.

No doubt some of this censure is due to the shadow that has been cast over public opinion about all public sector activity during the last decade. The last two presidents of the United States have been elected on "less-government" platforms embellished with overtly antigovernment rhetoric. Scorn for the capabilities and dedication of the public servant has become commonplace. It is little wonder that in such a climate skepticism should be voiced about the effectiveness of health departments.

Although some of the criticism aimed at health departments may be deserved, the committee believes that the future of public health depends on redefining and restoring the role of health agencies at all levels of government to a position of respect. Clearly, re-valuing the public sector responsibility for health will require strategies to respond to sound criticisms and improve the effectiveness of health departments. But it also requires a change in the American dialogue about the necessity and worth of public sector activity—of governance.

In summary, the committee defines the *organizational framework* of public health to encompass both activities undertaken within the formal structure of government and the associated efforts of private and voluntary organizations and individuals.

THE ROLE OF GOVERNMENT IN PUBLIC HEALTH

"The state is a facilitator . . . a convener . . . maybe a funder."

"I believe government ought to be involved in all areas where people can't do for themselves, health included."

"Who is responsible for planning health care delivery? Who will provide leadership?"

"Public health can lead the way . . . can get the ear of the decision-makers. Politics is going to be a part of this; there's no way around it."

"The overall responsibility of government is to assure the public that the environment is safe. Rules and regulations must be designed to serve that goal."

"A big job of government is to collect information, to figure out what causes the problem."

In general, Americans are skeptical about the role of government. Concern for individual rights shapes the public philosophy and attitudes of policymakers and ordinary citizens alike. (Heclo, 1986) From this perspective, society is made up of individual persons with "inalienable rights." The purpose of government is to protect those rights and ensure the basic conditions necessary for their exercise—civil order, a free market, and equal individual opportunity. Government, in other words, ensures that the basic means to the good life are available, but it refrains from specifying what the content of that life should be or how individuals should behave, except to prevent them from infringing on the rights of others.

This mainstream perspective is tempered somewhat by another long-standing tradition in American political philosophy, rooted in concern for the community as a whole. This view emphasizes the social ties that bind people together, including the values they share. It sees government as a facilitator of the social bond and the policy process as a means of defining

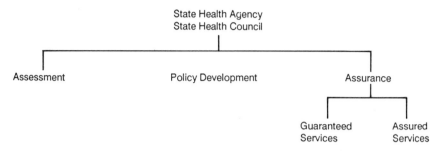

FIGURE 2.2   Relationship between government functions.

positive goals and taking concerted action. These two themes are reflected in the history of American governance. In general, the philosophy of limited government implied by a concern for individual rights has prevailed. But the theme of positive values and community effort has persisted, and deliberate government steps to combat acknowledged social ills have become increasingly acceptable to most Americans, remaining so even during the renewed stress on individualism in recent years.

Given the caution with which government action is approached in the United States, it is appropriate that the role envisioned for government in the mission of public health should be somewhat limited. Nevertheless, within this limited scope fall a number of key functions that fulfill values implied by each of the two philosophical traditions. If the range of government action is narrow, the substance is no less crucial to the well-being of the American people.

THE FUNCTIONS OF GOVERNMENT IN PUBLIC HEALTH

The committee sees the government role in public health as made up of three functions: assessment, policy development, and assurance (see Figures 2.2 and 2.3). These functions correspond to the major phases of public problem-solving: identification of problems, mobilization of necessary effort and resources, and assurance that vital conditions are in place and that crucial services are received.

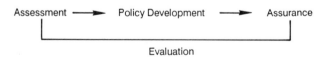

FIGURE 2.3   The government role in health.

Assessment

Under this heading are all the activities involved in the concept of community diagnosis, such as surveillance, identifying needs, analyzing the causes of problems, collecting and interpreting data, case-finding, monitoring and forecasting trends, research, and evaluation of outcomes.

Assessment is inherently a public function because policy formulation, in order to be legitimate, is expected to take in all relevant available information and to be based on objective factors—to the extent possible. Private sector entities are expected to have self-interests. Therefore the information they generate, while frequently quite useful to the policy process, is not judged by its fairness. In contrast, although public agencies in practice do not always weigh all sides of a question, in principle they are obligated to do so.

Moreover, public decisions take place in the context of limited resources. Society cannot do everything it would like to do or with the intensity it might prefer. Thus trade-offs among competing uses of resources are necessary. The wisdom, justice, and perceived legitimacy of public decisions are crucially affected by the quality of the information on which they are based. A function of government is to provide a central mechanism by means of which competing proposals can be assessed equitably.

In addition, the government has an important responsibility to develop a broader base of knowledge in order to ensure that policy is not driven by purely short-range issues constrained by current knowledge. Public sector assessment activities should include supporting and conducting research into fundamental determinants of health—behavioral, environmental, biological, and socioeconomic—as well as monitoring health status and trends.

The assessment function facilitates good decisions in both the private and public sectors. Since assessment seldom has its own constituency, however, it is often starved for resources. A fully developed assessment function is an absolutely essential part of the ideal public health system, and it is one that the committee believes to be in large measure attainable.

Policy Development

Policy formulation takes place as the result of interactions among a wide range of public and private organizations and individuals. It is the process by which society makes decisions about problems, chooses goals and the proper means to reach them, handles conflicting views about what should be done, and allocates resources. Government provides overall guidance in this process. In contrast to private entities, it alone has the power to give binding answers. Therefore, although it joins with the private sector to arrive at decisions, government has a special obligation to ensure that the public interest is served by whatever measures are adopted. As with other governmental entities, the public health agency bears this responsibility.

Examples of the governmental policy development role include planning and priority-setting; policy leadership and advocacy; convening, negotiating, and brokering; mobilizing resources; training constituency building and provision of public information; and encouragement of private and public sector action through incentives and persuasion.

The public health agency's special role in policy development means it must pay attention to the quality of the process itself, in addition to that of particular decisions. It must raise crucial questions that no one else raises; initiate communication with all affected parties, including the public-at-large; consider long-range issues in addition to crises; plan ahead as well as react; speak on behalf of persons and groups who have difficulty being heard in the process; build bridges between fragmented concerns; and strive for fairness and balance.

The public health agency should be equipped for this role by its technical knowledge and professional expertise. Used judiciously, the knowledge base of public health tempers the excesses of partisan politics and makes for more just decisions. Technical knowledge will have the best effect, however, when used in the context of a positive appreciation for the democratic political process, by professionals who are politically as well as technically astute.

Assurance

A core public sector function is to make sure that necessary services are provided to reach agreed upon goals, either by encouraging private sector action, by requiring it, or by providing services directly.

The assurance function in public health involves seeing to the implementation of legislative mandates as well as maintaining statutory responsibilities. It includes developing adequate responses to crises and supporting crucial services that have worked well for so long that they are now taken for granted. It includes regulation of services and products provided in both the private and public sectors, as well as maintaining accountability to the people by setting objectives and reporting on progress. Assurance implies the maintenance of a level of service needed to attain an intended impact or outcome that is achievable given the resources and techniques available.

Carrying out the assurance function requires the exercise of authority. This is not a responsibility that can be delegated to the private sector. Members of society expect government to make certain that they enjoy at least adequate safety and security. The public health agency must be able to exercise authority consistent with fulfilling citizens' expectations and must account to them for its actions with equal energy.

As a part of the assurance function, in the interest of justice public health agencies should guarantee certain health services. Such a guarantee expresses a measurable public commitment to each member of society. In operational terms, this implies guaranteeing both that the services are available (present somewhere in the community) and, in the case of services to individuals, that the costs will be borne by the government for those unable to afford them. When these services are not and cannot be present in the larger community, it is the public health agency's responsibility to provide them directly.

Such a guarantee reflects a community consensus that access to certain health services is necessary to maintain our notion of a decent society. A guarantee acts as a barrier to service cuts in hard times, which tend to fall on the must vulnerable. Such a step also serves as a stimulus to improvement, as has happened in the case of public education, where community efforts have moved from ensuring universal coverage to enriching the quality of the service.

The committee notes the examples set by the State of Michigan, which has guaranteed by law prenatal care to every woman in the state, and by San Diego County, California, which has a county-funded system making available acute care to all medically indigent adults.

In recent years a competitive market approach to the provision of health services has been advanced as the potential solution to ills that plague the U.S. health system, cost inflation in particular. While recognizing the existence of competition in service delivery, the committee believes that the responsibilities outlined above must be exercised by government in order to ensure basic capacity throughout the system.

The government role in public health provides the necessary context for private sector activity. Government is responsible for striving to achieve a balance between the two great concerns in the American public philosophy: individual liberty and free enterprise on the one hand, just and equitable action for the good of the community on the other.

Many times during the study, the committee heard public health defined as "what the market can't or won't do." Such comments usually refer to particular services and activities for which the market offers inadequate incentives, such as primary health care for those who can't pay or public services such as air pollution control. The committee acknowledges the existence of this residual view of public health, but observes that to define public health as what the market can't or won't do implies a passive or indifferent public sector and suggests that what the market can't do is not worth the concerned attention of society. On the contrary, recognition of the shortcomings or indifference of the market with respect to certain crucial needs should act as the rationale and catalyst for government action. Such action can take various forms: encouraging the development of private sector financial incentives where none now exist, so that, for example, the care of the uninsured could be made attractive to private providers; building helping relationships between public and private personnel, as when public health nurses complement the work of private practice physicians serving indigent patients; or imposing sanctions for failure to abide by regulatory requirements. Where incentives cannot be mobilized, the public health agency must and should provide necessary services directly.

At any level of government, the public sector responsibility for the health of the people must have a focal point in one agency charged with taking the lead in assuring that necessary obligations are fulfilled. Although it may sometimes be appropriate for public health-related responsibilities to be allocated among more than one public agency in addition to the health department, the committee believes that fulfilling the assurance function adequately requires that there be one place of ultimate responsibility and accountability.

Figure 2.4 presents a schematic diagram that illustrates the relative roles of the government and the private sectors in assuring and guaranteeing public health services.

STATE, LOCAL, AND FEDERAL ROLES IN PUBLIC HEALTH

The framers of the Constitution of the United States understood that the "federal" system of government they created was not an end in itself but a means to distribute power among the national government and those of the states. (Grodzins, 1985) They provided for state delegation of specific powers to the national government. All other powers were reserved to the states, and to this day states and the central government—that which we now call "federal"—share functions and power.

States in turn are the architects of local governments, of which today there are a bewildering array, including counties, municipalities, townships, school districts, and special districts. The overall three-level system of federal, state, and local governments includes over 80,000 governmental units. As one observer notes:

The enormous complexity of this system . . . suggests that it is impossible to have enough data to operate within it in a consistently rational fashion. . . . [E]fforts to orchestrate dramatic change . . . are bound to fall short of expectations. . . . (O'Toole, 1985)

Relationships among the many parties in the system are not hierarchical, but a matter of give and take. "Different governments need each other, and bargaining . . . is the norm." (O'Toole, 1985) Nor are patterns of interaction static; rather they are constantly changing. In addition, the distribution of functions and responsibilities among levels of government varies greatly from place to place, and many functions are shared, often in complex ways. Nevertheless, some broad generalizations can be made.

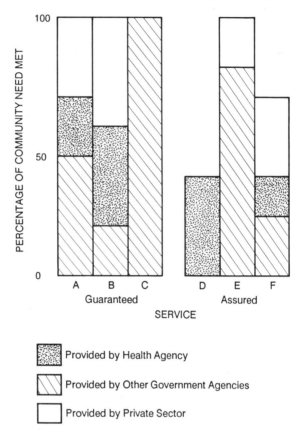

FIGURE 2.4 Government role in assured and guaranteed services. Each column shows how need for a specific health service may be met. The percentage of need met for each service by the three sources will vary by service and by location. In all cases 100 percent of need for Guaranteed Services should be met. While meeting 100 percent of the need for Assured Services should remain the ultimate public health objective, only part of this need will be met at the present time because of resource constraints or other limitations.

State Governments

Under the Constitution, the states are the repositories of powers not specifically delegated to the federal government. They have the primary responsibility for the well-being—including the health—of their citizens, and have exercised their powers over the years in a multitude of ways. They are the constitutional source of local government authority and can delegate broad powers over health matters to county and municipal governments.

The marked expansion of federal activism beginning in the Franklin D. Roosevelt presidency and the huge increase in intergovernmental fiscal transfer programs during the 1960s and 1970s added greatly to state responsibilities without removing existing ones. At the same time, because conventional policy wisdom was critical of state administrative capability and skeptical of some states' willingness to fulfill national priorities, many federal funding programs bypassed state governments entirely. Today, despite increased state activity and despite considerable efforts in the states to reform governance processes, according to the Advisory Commission on Intergovernmental Relations, "it does seem that improvements in state governmental performance have not been matched by a commensurate increase in their role as independent polities and policymakers." (Advisory Commission on Intergovernmental Relations, 1985)

Yet their constitutional role and accumulated responsibilities guarantee that states will continue to be the "pivotal actors in our federal system." (Advisory Commission on Intergovernmental Relations, 1985) The recent decline in federal activism and growing tolerance for state- and local-level diversity provide an opening for states to demonstrate their effectiveness.

This context sets the stage for asserting the central position of the states in public health. The key ingredients of this role include:

• Statewide assessment, policy development, and assurance. It is the state's responsibility to see that functions and services necessary to address the mission of public health are in place throughout the state. This can be done by encouraging, providing assistance to, and/or requiring local governments or private providers to perform certain of these functions. The state may also elect to provide certain services directly.

• Designating a lead agency for public health in the state (the place of ultimate responsibility) to fulfill the functions of assessment, policy development, and assurance. In most cases this will be the state health department, which has the obligation—and should have the authority—to ensure that important public health policy goals are being met, even when their implementation has been assigned to another entity.

State primacy in public health presents an opportunity for the entire nation to benefit by learning from evaluations of innovations and variations in public health programs at the state level.

Federal Government

Two developments since the founding period laid the groundwork for the enormous expansion of federal government health activity in modern times. First, the Supreme Court decision in *McCulloch v. Maryland* set out the doctrine of implied powers, which expanded the potential powers of the national government beyond those specifically delegated in the Constitution to those reasonably implied by the delegated powers. (*McCulloch v. Maryland,* 1819) Second, the passage in 1913 of the Sixteenth Amendment, authorizing a national income tax, substantially expanded the federal revenue-raising capability.

The commerce clause, interpreted under the doctrine of implied powers, and the power to tax for the general welfare under the Constitution have been the primary bases for much of national government health activity. Under the commerce clause, the Congress has the power to regulate commerce affecting more than one state, including health aspects of commerce. Federal grants-in-aid to states and localities in support of the general welfare have enabled the federal government to influence state- and local-health activity in line with national priorities. In addition, the federal government provides technical advice and assistance to states.

A long era of expansion in the federal role began in the 1930s and continued through the Great Society period of the 1960s. During the following decade the tide turned, and a nationwide redirection of emphasis emerged. This trend has decreased the federal presence in health, among other policy areas, and resulted in increasing reliance on state- and local-level activity and funding.

Despite the relative deemphasis on national government action, the federal role remains crucial. A primary activity is overall health policy development for the nation, including a variety of efforts to focus nationwide attention on major public health problems and encourage action on the part of other levels of government and of private groups. Such efforts may appropriately include provision of funds, but the potential for federal health policy leadership extends far beyond what can or should be expressed in dollars.

Federal leadership in public health issues is particularly critical if national scientific and professional expertise is to play its proper role in the policy process, offsetting the influence of special interests that tend to be especially decisive in smaller-scale public affairs. Public health's knowledge base is the core of what it has to offer to protect the health of the American people, and this knowledge depends on national government advocacy in order to function most effectively.

The federal government also plays an irreplaceable role in the development of national health data and in the conduct of research.

Local Governments

The vast numbers, overlapping jurisdictions, and varying authority of local governments make generalization difficult. Service responsibilities and fiscal capabilities are heterogeneous, and often the unit obligated to provide a service is not responsible for its financial support. From the public health perspective, perhaps the central problem is that our three-level model of government, placing basic responsibility for the people's health at the state level, does not fit well with the reality that health services must be delivered locally.

In constitutional law, local governments are clearly creatures of the states. Still, tradition and politics have combined to give the locals a strong voice in intergovernmental affairs, and in most states public health authority is substantially decentralized. In addition, in recent years many local governments have dealt directly with the federal government in connection with federal grants-in-aid and revenue sharing.

Given this context, the strengths of local governments for the provision of public health are (1) to serve as a governmental presence at the local level, ensuring each citizen's access to the security, protection, and authority of government; (2) to provide a mechanism for implementation and integration of a complex array of needed services; (3) to perform these functions on the basis of both professional and community-specific knowledge and in line with community values to the extent that they are consistent with the maintenance of individual rights; and (4) to convey information on local needs, priorities, and program effects to the state and national levels.

THE PUBLIC AND PRIVATE SECTORS IN PUBLIC HEALTH

In the history of public health the line between public and private responsibilities has never been hard and fast. It has shifted and blurred in response to changes in public health knowledge and in political agendas. In many respects, the varying points at which the boundary was drawn during the evolution of public health became de facto definitions that continue today to shape the way in which it is perceived.

Early public health activities, focused on combating and preventing epidemics, were mainly matters of sanitary engineering and environmental hygiene, because illness was believed to be associated with "dirt." Private physicians were among a wide range of active participants in the early citizen hygiene associations that joined with governments in these efforts. (Duffy, 1979) During this period, public health was aimed at preventing illness by improving living conditions, and care of individual patients was left to private physicians. With the discovery of bacteria and the development of immunization techniques, however, disease prevention could no longer be so easily defined solely as a communitywide affair. The line between prevention and treatment began to fade, and the domains of public health and private medicine could no longer be easily separated. This development created a certain amount of tension between the two that has never fully been resolved. (Rosenkrantz, 1974; Duffy, 1979; Starr, 1982) Given its continuing need for medical expertise, public health has struggled ever since to assert a positive role for itself and to maintain an accord with the medical profession.

In modern times the focus of tension has shifted again, ironically in the direction of bringing the medical care of individual patients more strongly within the purview of public health than ever before. Increasingly, health departments have become "providers of last resort" for uninsured patients and those Medicaid patients rejected by or simply beyond the reach of private providers and institutions. Once immersed exclusively in population-wide and community-based efforts, health departments have rapidly become de facto family doctors for millions of Americans.

While aware that there are complex reasons behind these developments, the committee does not believe that the ideal public health system is defined in the way in which Robert Frost once defined "home"—as that place where, "when you have to go there, they have to take you in." Clearly, the line between community-based and individual strategies in disease prevention and health promotion cannot be simply drawn. It is evident, however, that the failure to define a positive role for the public sector in public health is producing what one observer of U.S. attempts to deal with AIDS has called a "crisis of authority." (Fox, 1986)

As the place where the health buck stops, the official health agency at a given level of government must be the locus of decision-making to assure that necessary functions and services are in place. The public sector is also the most appropriate provider of health services that are poorly handled in the market. But the direct provision by health departments of personal health care to patients who are unwanted by the private sector absorbs so much of the limited resources available to public health—money, human resources, energy, time, and attention—that the price is higher than it appears. Maintenance functions—those communitywide public services that are truly ill-suited to the private sector—become stunted because they cannot compete, and key functions such as assessment and policy development wither because they are not seen as life-and-death matters.

In the ideal U.S. health system, given our traditions and values, most personal medical care, regardless of payment status, would be provided by the private sector. In the same ideal, public health would emphasize specialized personal health services uniquely needed for fulfilling the assurance function of the public health mission. The committee notes that care of the poor and the uninsured has indeed become an issue in the private sector, in the form of concern over "uncompensated care." The slow starvation of classic public health activities offers an additional compelling reason for finding what one public health official interviewed in the study called a "medical home" for poor Americans, one that makes sense in terms of patient needs and professional capabilities, not simply a place that has to take them in.

THE BASIC SERVICES OF PUBLIC HEALTH

The potential list of basic public health services is diverse. Although the practice of public health can be traced back to the ancient Greek interest in the relationship between environmental factors and disease (Ellencweig and Yoshpe, 1984), over the centuries a wide range of notions has come to be more or less accepted under the public health umbrella. To environmental health, preventive medicine, epidemiology, and disease control have been added such disparate concerns as primary medical care, advocacy, school health, crisis response, family planning, care of the poor, dental care, licensure and certification, mental health, and home health care, to name only some of the topics raised in the committee's conversations with practitioners, clients, and others.

A basic service is one that **fulfills society's interest in assuring conditions in which people can be healthy,** to refer back to the defined mission of public health. It should be emphasized again that assuring the presence of these services is a governmental function, but their provision is a responsibility shared by both public and private sectors.

There are several possible ways to consider the issue of basics; combined, they may provide workable guidance for policy-making.

One aspect of the issue is the substantive areas that make up the commitment. Health activities can be grouped under three broad headings: personal health services, or medical care; environmental measures; and education. Certainly the governmental commitment, the public health mission, requires attention to all three of these substantive areas.

Another aspect of the question "What are the basics?" has to do with shared objectives. *Model Standards: A Guide for Community Preventive Health Services* is a set of standards for organizing local health services. It was developed by the American Public Health Association, the national organizations for state health officers, county health officials, local health officers, and the U.S. Public Health Service. It has demonstrated that commitment to "a governmental presence at the local level" can be carried beyond vague generalities and translated into specifics about what constitutes an *acceptable* effort. This document lists 34 categories of public services that should be available at the local level. (American Public Health Association et al., 1985; see also Appendix C)

The 1990 *Objectives for the Nation* of the U.S. Public Health Service also encourage conscious and systematic assessment of need, setting of targets, monitoring of progress, and evaluation of outcome to promote health and prevent disease. It is important to set goals and report to the public on progress toward them even when their accomplishment cannot be assured. (U.S. Department of Health and Human Services, 1980; see also Appendix C) The document targets 18 health problems with objectives for preventing them. Subsequent documents by the Public Health Service have measured the nation's and states' progress toward meeting these goals.

Finally, there is the issue of whether the idea of basic services suggests a minimum set, full provision of which should be guaranteed by government to all members of society. The next two chapters will paint the picture of a public health system that is incredibly diverse. The fact that there is considerable inconsistency among states and in local areas as to existing services in government health agencies raises the question of whether certain services should be available everywhere as a matter of justice. Clearly, although there is widespread agreement about the value of many so-called basic services, in practice the trade-offs made necessary by limited resources means that some basics are sacrificed to still higher priorities, some of them perhaps outside the health area entirely. Are there some public health services that should never be sacrificed, no matter what? Does a governmental obligation to assure conditions in which people can be healthy extend to *requiring* certain of these conditions?

The committee believes that the answer to these questions is "Yes." In Michigan, prenatal care is guaranteed to every resident, with support provided for those unable to pay. The Michigan example does not imply that every state should guarantee prenatal care; it does imply that every state should ask itself explicitly what services are so crucial that access to their benefits ought to be guaranteed, and make good its obligation by providing the required resources when other providers can't or won't.

To sum up, the answer to the question "What are the basics?" of government's responsibility for the people's health encompasses the following elements: assuring a substantive core of activities, assuring adequacy of means and methods, establishing objectives, and providing guarantees. In the ideal health system, the substance of basic services will entail adequate personal health care for all members of the community, the education of individuals about healthy life-styles and the education of the community-at-large, the control of communicable disease, and the control of environmental hazards—biological, chemical, social, and physical. Explicit priorities will be set in each community and at each level of government so that clear objectives guide organized community efforts. And governments will hold themselves accountable to the people by undertaking to guarantee certain services to all as a matter of justice.

REFERENCES

Advisory Commission on Intergovernmental Relations. 1985. *The Question of State Government Capability.* Advisory Commission on Intergovernmental Relations, Washington, D.C.

American Public Health Association, Association of State and Territorial Health Officials, National Association of County Health Officials, U.S. Conference of Local Health Officials, Department of Health and Human Services, Public Health Service. 1985. *Model Standards: A Guide for Community Preventive Health Services.* American Public Health Association, Washington, D.C.

Beauchamp, Dan. 1976. "Public Health as Social Justice." *Inquiry* 13:3–14.

Duffy, John. 1979. "The American Medical Profession and Public Health: From Support to Ambivalence." *Bulletin of the History of Medicine* 53(Spring):1:1–22.

Ellencweig, Avi Yacar, and Ruthellen B. Yoshpe. 1984. "Definition of Public Health." *Public Health Review* 12:65–78.

Fox, Daniel M. 1986. "AIDS and the American Health Policy: The History and Prospects of a Crisis of Authority." *The Milbank Quarterly* 64(Spring Supplement):1:7–33.

Grodzins, Morton. 1985. "The Federal System." Pp. 43–50 in *American Intergovernmental Relations,* Lawrence J. O'Toole, Jr., ed. Congressional Quarterly Press, Washington, D.C.

Hanlon, G., and J. Pickett. 1984. *Public Health Administration and Practice.* Times Mirror/ Mosby.

Heclo, Hugh. 1986. "Reaganism and the Search for a Public Philosophy." In *Perspectives on the Reagan Years,* John L. Palmer, ed. Urban Institute Press, Washington, D.C.

McCulloch v. Maryland 17 U.S.(4 Wheaton)316 (1819).

O'Toole, Jr., Lawrence J. 1985. "American Intergovernmental Relations: Concluding Thoughts," Lawrence J. O'Toole, Jr., ed. *American Intergovernmental Relations.* Congressional Quarterly Press, Washington, D.C.

Robbins, Anthony. 1985. "Public Health in the Next Decade." *Journal of Public Health Policy* 6(4):440–46.

Rosenkrantz, Barbara Gutmann. 1972. *Public Health and the State: Changing Views in Massachusetts, 1842–1936.* Harvard University Press, Cambridge.

Rosenkrantz, Barbara Gutmann. 1974. "Cart Before Horse: Theory, Practice and Professional Image in American Public Health, 1870–1920." *Journal of the History of Medicine* (January):55–73.

Starr, Paul. 1982. *The Social Transformation of American Medicine.* Basic Books, New York.

Terris, Miller. 1985. "The Public Health Profession." *Journal of Public Health Policy* 6:1:7–14.

Terris, Milton. 1986. "Preventing the Final Epidemic: The Role of the American Public Health Association and the International Epidemiological Association." *Journal of Public Health Policy* 7(18:7–11).

U.S. Department of Health and Human Services, Public Health Service. 1980. *Promoting Health Preventing Disease: Objectives for the Nation.* U.S. Department of Health and Human Services, Washington, D.C.

3

A History of the
Public Health System

In Chapter 1, the committee found that the current public health system must play a critical role in handling major threats to the public health, but that this system is currently in disarray. Chapter 2 explained the committee's ideal for the public health system—how it should be arranged for handling current and future threats to health. In this chapter the history of the existing public health system is briefly described. This history is intended to provide some perspective on how protection of citizens from health threats came to be a public responsibility and on how the public health system came to be in its current state.

HISTORY

During the past 150 years, two factors have shaped the modern public health system: first, the growth of scientific knowledge about sources and means of controlling disease; second, the growth of public acceptance of disease control as both a possibility and a public responsibility. In earlier centuries, when little was known about the causes of disease, society tended to regard illness with a degree of resignation, and few public actions were taken. As understanding of sources of contagion and means of controlling disease became more refined, more effective interventions against health threats were developed. Public organizations and agencies were formed to employ newly discovered interventions against health threats. As scientific knowledge grew, public authorities expanded to take on new tasks, including sanitation, immunization, regulation, health education, and personal health care. (Chave, 1984; Fee, 1987)

The link between science, the development of interventions, and organization of public authorities to employ interventions was increased public understanding of and social commitment to enhancing health. The growth of a public system for protecting health depended both on scientific discovery and social action. Understanding of disease made public measures to alleviate pain and suffering possible, and social values about the worthiness of this goal made public measures feasible. The history of the public health system is a history of bringing knowledge and values together in the public arena to shape an approach to health problems.

BEFORE THE EIGHTEENTH CENTURY

Throughout recorded history, epidemics such as the plague, cholera, and smallpox evoked sporadic public efforts to protect citizens in the face of a dread disease. Although epidemic disease was often considered a sign of poor moral and spiritual condition, to be mediated through prayer and piety, some public effort was made to contain the epidemic spread of specific disease through isolation of the ill and quarantine of travelers. In the late seventeenth century, several European cities appointed public authorities to adopt and enforce isolation and quarantine measures (and to report and record deaths from the plague). (Goudsblom, 1986)

THE EIGHTEENTH CENTURY

By the eighteenth century, isolation of the ill and quarantine of the exposed became common measures for containing specified contagious diseases. Several American port cities adopted rules for trade quarantine and isolation of the sick. In 1701 Massachusetts passed laws for isolation of smallpox patients and for ship quarantine as needed. (After 1721, inoculation with material from smallpox scabs was also accepted as an effective means of containing this disease once the threat of an epidemic was declared.) By the end of the eighteenth century, several cities, including Boston, Philadelphia, New York, and Baltimore, had established permanent councils to enforce quarantine and isolation rules. (Hanlon and Pickett, 1984) These eighteenth-century initiatives reflected new ideas about both the cause and meaning of disease. Diseases were seen less as natural effects of the human condition and more as potentially controllable through public action.

Also in the eighteenth century, cities began to establish voluntary general hospitals for the physically ill and public institutions for the care of the mentally ill. Finally, physically and mentally ill dependents were cared for by their neighbors in local communities. This practice was made official in England with the adoption of the 1601 Poor Law and continued in the

American colonies. (Grob, 1966; Starr, 1982) By the eighteenth century, several communities had reached a size that demanded more formal arrangements for care of their ill than Poor Law practices. The first American voluntary hospitals were established in Philadelphia in 1752 and in New York in 1771. The first public mental hospital was established in Williamsburg, Virginia in 1773. (Turner, 1977)

THE NINETEENTH CENTURY: THE GREAT SANITARY AWAKENING

The nineteenth century marked a great advance in public health. "The great sanitary awakening" (Winslow, 1923)—the identification of filth as both a cause of disease and a vehicle of transmission and the ensuing embrace of cleanliness—was a central component of nineteenth-century social reforms. Sanitation changed the way society thought about health. Illness came to be seen as an indicator of poor social and environmental conditions, as well as poor moral and spiritual conditions. Cleanliness was embraced as a path both to physical and moral health. Cleanliness, piety, and isolation were seen to be compatible and mutually reinforcing measures to help the public resist disease. At the same time, mental institutions became oriented toward "moral treatment" and cure.

Sanitation also changed the way society thought about public responsibility for citizen's health. Protecting health became a social responsibility. Disease control continued to focus on epidemics, but the manner of controlling turned from quarantine and isolation of the individual to cleaning up and improving the common environment. And disease control shifted from reacting to intermittent outbreaks to continuing measures for prevention. With sanitation, public health became a societal goal and protecting health became a public activity.

The Sanitary Problem

With increasing urbanization of the population in the nineteenth century, filthy environmental conditions became common in working class areas, and the spread of disease became rampant. In London, for example, smallpox, cholera, typhoid, and tuberculosis reached unprecedented levels. It was estimated that as many as 1 person in 10 died of smallpox. More than half the working class died before their fifth birthday. Meanwhile, "In the summers of 1858 and 1859 the Thames stank so badly as to rise 'to the height of an historic event . . . for months together the topic almost monopolized the public prints'." (Winslow, 1923) London was not alone in this dilemma. In New York, as late as 1865, "the filth and garbage accumulate in the streets to the depth sometimes of two or three feet." In a 2-week survey of tenements in the sixteenth ward of New York, inspectors found more than 1,200 cases of smallpox and more than 2,000 cases of typhus. (Winslow, 1923) In Massachusetts in 1850, deaths from tuberculosis were 300 per 100,000 population, and infant mortality was about 200 per 1,000 live births. (Hanlon and Pickett, 1984)

Earlier measures of isolation and quarantine during specific disease outbreaks were clearly inadequate in an urban society. It was simply impossible to isolate crowded slum dwellers or quarantine citizens who could not afford to stop working. (Wohl, 1983) It also became clear that diseases were not just imported from other shores, but were internally generated. "The belief that epidemic disease posed only occasional threats to an otherwise healthy social order was shaken by the industrial transformation of the nineteenth century." (Fee, 1987) Industrialization, with its overburdened workforce and crowded dwellings, produced both a population more susceptible to disease and conditions in which disease was more easily transmitted. (Wohl, 1983) Urbanization, and the resulting concentration of filth, was considered in and of itself a cause of disease. "In the absence of specific etiological concepts, the social and physical conditions which accompanied urbanization were considered equally responsible for the impairment of vital bodily functions and premature death." (Rosenkrantz, 1972)

At the same time, public responsibility for the health of the population became more acceptable and fiscally possible. In earlier centuries, disease was more readily identified as only the plight of the impoverished and immoral. The plague had been regarded as a disease of the poor; the wealthy could retreat to country estates and, in essence, quarantine themselves. In the urbanized nineteenth century, it became obvious that the wealthy could not escape contact with the poor. "Increasingly, it dawned upon the rich that they could not ignore the plight of the poor; the proximity of gold coast and slum was too close." (Goudsblom, 1986) And the spread of contagious disease in these cities was not selective. Almost all families lost children to diphtheria, smallpox, or other infectious diseases. Because of the the deplorable social and environmental conditions and the constant threat of disease spread, diseases came to be considered an indicator of a societal problem as well as a personal problem. "Poverty and disease could no longer be treated simply as individual failings." (Fee, 1987) This view included not only contagious disease, but mental illness as well. Insanity came to be viewed at least in part as a societal failing, caused by physical, moral, and social tensions.

The Development of Public Activities in Health

Edwin Chadwick, a London lawyer and secretary of the Poor Law Commission in 1838, is one of the most recognized names in the sanitary reform movement. Under Chadwick's authority, the commission conducted studies of the life and health of the London working class in 1838 and that of the entire country in 1842. The report of these studies, *General Report on the*

Sanitary Conditions of the Labouring Population of Great Britain, "was a damning and fully documented indictment of the appalling conditions in which masses of the working people were compelled to live, and die, in the industrial towns and rural areas of the Kingdom." (Chave, 1984) Chadwick documented that the average age at death for the gentry was 36 years; for the tradesmen, 22 years; and for the laborers, only 16 years. (Hanlon and Pickett, 1984) To remedy the situation, Chadwick proposed what came to be known as the "sanitary idea." His remedy was based on the assumption that diseases are caused by foul air from the decomposition of waste. To remove disease, therefore, it was necessary to build a drainage network to remove sewage and waste. Further, Chadwick proposed that a national board of health, local boards in each district, and district medical officers be appointed to accomplish this goal. (Chave, 1984)

Chadwick's report was quite controversial, but eventually many of his suggestions were adopted in the Public Health Act of 1848. The report, which influenced later developments in public health in England and the United States, documented the extent of disease and suffering in the population, promoted sanitation and engineering as means of controlling disease, and laid the foundation for public infrastructure for combating and preventing contagious disease.

In the United States, similar studies were taking place. Inspired in part by Chadwick, local sanitary surveys were conducted in several cities. The most famous of these was a survey conducted by Lemuel Shattuck, a Massachusetts bookseller and statistician. His *Report of the Massachusetts Sanitary Commission* was published in 1850. Shattuck collected vital statistics on the Massachusetts population, documenting differences in morbidity and mortality rates in different localities. He attributed these differences to urbanization, specifically the foulness of the air created by decay of waste in areas of dense population, and to immoral life-style. He showed that the poor living conditions in the city threatened the entire community. "Even those persons who attempted to maintain clean and decent homes were foiled in their efforts to resist diseases if the behavior of others invited the visitation of epidemics." (Rosenkrantz, 1972)

Shattuck considered immorality an important influence on susceptibility to ill health—and in fact drunkenness and sloth did often lead to poor health in the slums—but he believed that these conditions were threatening to all. Further, Shattuck determined that those most likely to be affected by disease were also those who, either through ignorance or lack of concern, failed to take personal responsibility for cleanliness and sanitation of their area. (Rosenkrantz, 1972) Consequently, he argued that the city or the state had to take responsibility for the environment. Shattuck's *Report of the Massachusetts Sanitary Commission* recommended, in its "Plan for a Sanitary Survey of the State," a comprehensive public health system for the state.

The report recommended, among other things, new census schedules; regular surveys of local health conditions; supervision of water supplies and waste disposal; special studies on specific diseases, including tuberculosis and alcoholism; education of health providers in preventive medicine; local sanitary associations for collecting and distributing information; and the establishment of a state board of health and local boards of health to enforce sanitary regulations. (Winslow, 1923; Rosenkrantz, 1972)

Shattuck's report was widely circulated after publication, but because of political upheaval at the time of release nothing was done. The report "fell flat from the printer's hand." In the years following the Civil War, however, the creation of special agencies became a more common method of handling societal problems. Massachusetts set up a state board of health in 1869. The creation of this board reflected more a trend of strengthened government than new knowledge about the causes and control of disease. Nevertheless, the type of data collected by Shattuck was used to justify the board. And the board relied on many of the recommendations of Shattuck's report for shaping a public health system. (Rosenkrantz, 1972; Hanlon and Pickett, 1984) Although largely ignored at the time of its release, Shattuck's report has come to be considered one of the most farsighted and influential documents in the history of the American public health system. Many of the principles and activities he proposed later came to be considered fundamental to public health. And Shattuck established the fundamental usefulness of keeping records and vital statistics.

Similarly, in New York, John Griscom published *The Sanitary Condition of the Labouring Population of New York* in 1848. This report eventually led to the establishment of the first public agency for health, the New York City Health Department, in 1866. During this same period, boards of health were established in Louisiana, California, the District of Columbia, Virginia, Minnesota, Maryland, and Alabama. (Fee, 1987; Hanlon and Pickett, 1984) By the end of the nineteenth century, 40 states and several local areas had established health departments.

Although the specific mechanisms of diseases were still poorly understood, collective action against contagious disease proved to be successful. For example, cholera was known to be a waterborne disease, but the precise agent of infection was not known at this time. The sanitary reform movement brought more water to cities in the mid-nineteenth century, through private contractors and eventually through reservoirs and municipal water supplies, but its usefulness did not depend primarily on its purity for consumption, but its availability for washing and fire protection. (Blake, 1956) Nonetheless, sanitary efforts of the New York Board of Health in 1866, including inspections, immediate case reporting, complaint investigations, evacuations, and disinfection of possessions and living quarters, kept an outbreak of cholera to a small number of cases. "The mildness of the epidemic was no more a stroke of good fortune, observers agreed, but the result of careful planning and hard work by the new health board." (Rosenberg, 1962) Cities without a public system for monitoring and combatting the disease fared far worse in the 1866 epidemic.

During this period, states also established more public institutions for care of the mentally ill. Dorothea Dix, a retired school teacher from Maine, is the most familiar name in the reform movement for care of the mentally ill. In the early nineteenth century, under Poor Law practices, communities that could not place their poor mentally ill citizens in more appropriate institutions put them in municipal jails and almshouses. Beginning in the middle of the century, Dix led a crusade to publicize the inhumane treatment mentally ill citizens were receiving in jails and campaigned for the establishment of more public institutions for care of the insane. In the nineteenth century, mental illness was considered a combination of inherited characteristics, medical problems, and social, intellectual, moral, and economic failures. It was believed, despite the prejudice that the poor and foreign-born were more likely to be mentally ill, that moral treatment in a humane social setting could cure mental illness. Dix and others argued that in the long run institutional care was cheaper for the community. The mentally ill could be treated and cured in an institution, making continuing public support unnecessary. Some 32 public institutions were established due to Dix's efforts. Although the practice of moral treatment proved to be less successful than hoped, the nineteenth-century social reform movement established the principle of state responsibility for the indigent mentally ill. (Grob, 1966; Foley and Sharfstein, 1983)

New ideas about causes of disease and about social responsibility stimulated the development of public health agencies and institutions. As environmental and social causes of diseases were identified, social action appeared to be an effective way to control diseases. When health was no longer simply an individual responsibility, it became necessary to form public boards, agencies, and institutions to protect the health of citizens. Sanitary and social reform provided the basis for the formation of public health organizations.

Public health agencies and institutions started at the local and state levels in the United States. Federal activities in health were limited to the Marine Hospital Service, a system of public hospitals for the care of merchant seamen. Because merchant seamen had no local citizenship, the federal government took on the responsibility of providing their health care. A national board of health, which was intended to take over the responsibilities of the Marine Hospital Service, was adopted in 1879, but, opposed by the Marine Hospital Service and many southern states, the board lasted only until 1883 (Anderson, 1985) Meanwhile, several state boards of health, state health departments, and local health departments had been established by the latter part of the nineteenth century. (Hanlon and Pickett, 1984)

LATE NINETEENTH CENTURY: ENTER BACTERIOLOGY

Another major set of developments in public health took place at the close of the nineteenth century. Rapid advances in scientific knowledge about causes and prevention of numerous diseases brought about tremendous changes in public health. Many major contagious diseases were brought under control through science applied to public health. Louis Pasteur, a French chemist, proved in 1877 that anthrax is caused by bacteria. By 1884, he had developed artificial immunization against the disease. During the following few years, discoveries of bacteriologic agents of disease were made in European and American laboratories for such contagious diseases as tuberculosis, diphtheria, typhoid, and yellow fever. (Winslow, 1923)

The identification of bacteria and the development of interventions such as immunization and water purification techniques provided a means of controlling the spread of disease and even of preventing disease. The germ theory of disease provided a sound scientific basis for public health. Public health measures continued to be focused predominantly on specific contagious diseases, but the means of controlling these diseases changed dramatically. Laboratory research identified exact causes and specific strategies for preventing specific diseases. For the first time, it was known that diseases had single, specific causes. Science also revealed that both the environment and people could be the agents of disease. During this period public agencies that had been developed to conduct and enforce sanitary measures refined their activities and expanded into laboratory science and epidemiology. Public responsibility for health came to include both environmental sanitation and individual health.

The Development of State and Local Health Department Laboratories

To develop and apply the new scientific knowledge, in the 1890s state and local health departments in the United States began to establish laboratories. The first were established in Massachusetts, as a cooperative venture between the State Board of Health and the Massachusetts Institute of Technology, and in New York City, as a part of the New York City Health Department. These were quickly followed by a state hygienic laboratory in Ann Arbor, Michigan, and a municipal public health laboratory in Providence. (Winslow, 1923)

These laboratories concentrated on improving sanitation through detection and control of bacteria in water systems. W. T. Sedgwick, consulting biologist for Massachusetts, was one of the most famous scientists in sanitation and bacteriologic research. In 1891 he identified the presence of fecal bacteria in water as the cause of typhoid fever and developed the first sewage treatment techniques. Sedgwick followed his research on typhoid with many similar investigations of epidemics. "With the relish of a good storyteller, Sedgwick would unravel a plot in which the villain was a bacterial organism; the victim, the unwitting public; the hero, sanitary hygiene brought to life through the application of scientific methods." (Rosenkrantz, 1972) In the 1890s, Sedgwick also conducted research on bacteria in milk and was one of the main spokesmen for restrictive rules on the handling and pasteurization of milk.

Laboratory research was also applied to diagnosis of disease in individuals. Theobald Smith, director of the pathology laboratory in the federal Bureau of Animal Industry, earned an international reputation for his identification of the causes of several diseases in animals and the development of techniques to produce artificial immunity against them. Later, as director of a state laboratory in Massachusetts, Smith developed vaccines, antitoxins, and diagnostic tests against such diseases as smallpox, meningitis, tuberculosis, and typhoid. He established the principle of using biological products to produce immunity to a specific disease in the individual and argued that research on the process of disease in the individual as well as the cause of disease in the environment was necessary to develop effective interventions. (Rosenkrantz, 1972)

In New York, the city health department laboratory also promoted diagnosis of contagious diseases in individuals. New York was one of the first health departments to begin producing antitoxins for physicians' use, and the department offered free laboratory analyses. (Starr, 1982) Hermann Biggs, pathologist and later commissioner of the New York City Health Department, suggested the application of bacteriology to detecting and controlling cholera. W. H. Park, another pathologist in the laboratory, introduced bacteriological diagnosis of diphtheria and production of diphtheria antitoxin. (Winslow, 1923)

The Successes of Bacteriology

Some of the comments of the time reveal the enthusiasm with which the public health workers embraced the new scientific foundation for their efforts. Scientific measures were seen as replacing earlier social, sanitary, moral, and religious reform measures to combat disease. Science was seen as a more effective means of achieving the same desirable social goals. Sedgwick declared, "before 1880 we knew nothing; after 1890 we knew it all; it was a glorious ten years." (Fee, 1987) Charles Chapin, superintendent of Health of Providence, Rhode Island, who published *Sources and Modes of Infection* in 1910, argued for strictly scientific measures of infectious disease control. Chapin believed that time spent on cleaning cities was wasted, that instead health officers should concentrate on controlling specific routes of disease transmission. "There was little more reason for health departments to assume responsibility for street cleaning and control of nuisances, . . . than 'that they should work for free transfers, cheaper commutation tickets, lower prices for coal, less shoddy in clothing or more rubber in rubbers. . . . '" (Rosenkrantz, 1972) Herbert Hill, director of the Division of Epidemiology of the Minnesota Board of Health, compared the new epidemiologist to a hunter seeking a sheep-killing wolf: "Instead of finding in the mountains and following inward from them, say, 500 different wolf trails, 499 of which must necessarily be wrong, the experienced hunter goes directly to the slaughtered sheep, finding there and following outward thence the only right trail . . . the one trail that is necessarily and inevitably the trail of the one actually guilty wolf." (Hill, as quoted by Fee, 1987)

The new methods of disease control were remarkably effective. For example, prior to 1908 17 American cities had death rates from typhoid fever of 30 or more per 100,000 population; 18 had death rates between 15 and 30 per 100,000. After water filtering systems were put in place, only 3 of the same cities had rates exceeding 15 per 100,000. (Winslow, 1923) In another example, the number of deaths from yellow fever in Havana dropped from 305 to 6 in a single year after a team of American military scientists led by Walter Reed identified mosquitoes as carriers of the yellow fever virus. (Winslow, 1923)

As public health became a scientific enterprise, it also became the province of experts. Prevention and control of disease were no longer tasks of common sense and social compassion, but of knowledge and expertise. Health reforms were guided by engineers, chemists, biologists, and physicians. And the health department gained stature as a source of scientific knowledge in health. It became clear that not only public and individual restraint were needed to control infectious disease, but also state agency epidemiologists and their laboratories were needed to direct the way. (Rosenkrantz, 1974)

EARLY TWENTIETH CENTURY: THE MOVE TOWARD PERSONAL CARE

Further Development of State and Local Health Agencies

In the early twentieth century, the role of the state and local public health departments expanded greatly. Although disease control was based on bacteriology, it became increasingly clear that individual persons were more often the source of disease transmission than things. "The work of the laboratory led the Board to define the existence and character of an increasing number of the most dangerous diseases and to provide medical means for their control." (Rosenkrantz, 1972) Identification and treatment of individual cases of disease were the next natural steps. Massachusetts, Michigan, and New York City began producing and dispensing antitoxins in the 1890s. Several states established disease registries. In 1907, Massachusetts passed a law requiring reporting of individual cases of 16 different diseases. Required reporting implied an obligation to treat. For example, reporting of cancer was later added to the list, and a cancer treatment program began in 1927.

It also became clear that providing immunizations and treating infectious diseases did not solve all health problems. Despite remarkable success in lowering death rates from typhoid, diphtheria, and other contagious diseases, considerable disability continued to exist in the population. There were still numerous diseases, such as tuberculosis, for which infectious agents were not clearly identified. Draft registration during World War I revealed that a substantial portion of the male population was either physically or mentally unfit for combat. (Fee, 1987) It also became clear that diseases, even those for which treatment was available, still predominantly affected the urban poor. Registration and analysis of disease showed that the highest rates of morbidity still occurred among children and the poor. On the premise that a healthier society could be built through health care for individuals, health departments expanded into clinical care and health education. In the early twentieth century, the New York and Baltimore health departments began offering home visits by public health nurses. New York established a campaign for education on tuberculosis. (Winslow, 1923) School health clinics were set up in Boston in 1894, New York in 1903, Rhode Island in 1906, and many other cities in subsequent years. (Bremner, 1971) Numerous local health agencies set up clinics to deal with tuberculosis and infant mortality. By 1915, there were more than 500 tuberculosis clinics and 538 baby clinics in America, predominantly run by city health departments. These clinics concentrated on providing medical care and health education. (Starr, 1982)

As public agencies moved into clinical care and education, the orientation of public health shifted from disease prevention to promotion of overall health. Epidemiology provided a scientific justification for health programs that had originated with social reforms. Public health once again became a task of promoting a healthy society. In the twentieth century, this goal was to be achieved through scientific analysis of disease, medical treatment of individuals, and education on healthy habits. In 1923, C. E. A. Winslow defined public health as the science of not only preventing contagious disease, but also of "prolonging life, and promoting physical health and efficiency." (Winslow, as quoted in Hanlon and Pickett, 1984)

The Growth of Federal Activities in Health

Federal activities in public health also expanded during the late nineteenth century and the early twentieth century. The National Hygienic Laboratory, established in 1887 in the Marine Hospital in Staten Island, New York, included divisions in chemistry, zoology, and pharmacology. In 1906, Congress passed the Food and Drug Act, which initiated controls on the manufacture, labeling, and sale of food. In 1912, the Marine Hospital Service was renamed the U.S. Public Health Service, and its director, the surgeon general, was granted more authority. Although early Public Health Service activities were modest, by 1918 they included administering physical and mental examinations of aliens, demonstration projects in rural health, and control and prevention of venereal diseases. (Hanlon and Pickett, 1984) In 1914, Congress enacted the Chamberlain–Kahn Act, which established the U.S. Interdepartmental Social Hygiene Board, a comprehensive venereal disease control program for the military, and provided funds for quarantine of infected civilians. (Brandt, 1985)

Federal activities also grew to include promoting programs for individual health and providing assistance to states for campaigns against specific health problems. The Children's Bureau was formed in 1912, and the first White House Conference on child health was held in 1919. (Hanlon and Pickett, 1984) The Sheppard–Towner Act of 1922 established the Federal Board of Maternity and Infant Hygiene, provided administrative funds to the Children's Bureau, and provided funds to states to establish programs in maternal and child health. This act was the first to establish direct federal funding of personal health services. In order to receive federal funds, states were required to develop a plan for providing nursing, home care, health education, and obstetric care to mothers in the state; to designate a state agency to administer the program; and to report on operations and expenditures of the program to the federal board. The Sheppard–Towner Act was the impetus for the federal practice of setting guidelines for public health programs and providing funding to states to implement programs meeting the guidelines. Although federally initiated, the programs were fully state-run. (Bremner, 1971) As the federal bureaucracy in health grew and programs requiring federal–state partnerships for health programs were developed, the need for expertise and leaders in public health increased at both the federal and state level.

MID-TWENTIETH CENTURY: FURTHER EXPANSION OF THE GOVERNMENTAL ROLE IN PERSONAL HEALTH

From the 1930s through the 1970s, local, state, and federal responsibilities in health continued to increase. The federal role in health also became more prominent. A strong federal government and a strong government role in ensuring social welfare were publicly supported social values of this era. From Roosevelt's New Deal in the 1930s through Johnson's Great Society of the 1960s, a federal role in services affecting the health and welfare of individual citizens became well established. The federal government and state and local health agencies took on greater roles in providing and planning health services, in health promotion and health education, and in financing health services. The agencies also continued and increased activities in environmental sanitation, epidemiology, and health statistics.

Federal Activities

Federal programs in disease control, research, and epidemiology expanded throughout the mid-twentieth century. In 1930, the National Hygienic Laboratory relocated to the Washington, D.C., area and was renamed the National Institute of Health (NIH). In 1937, the Institute greatly expanded its research functions to include the study and investigation of all diseases and related conditions and the National Cancer Institute was established as the first of the research institutes focused on particular diseases or health problems. By the 1970s NIH grew to include an Institute for Neurological and Communicative Disorders and Stroke, an Institute for Child Health and Human Development, an Institute for Environmental Health Sciences, and an Institute of Mental Health, among others. In 1938, Congress passed a second venereal disease control act, which provided federal funds to states for investigation and control of venereal diseases. In 1939, the Federal Security Agency, housing the Public Health Service and national programs in education and welfare, was established. The Public Health Service also continued to expand. During World War II, the Center for Disease Control was established, and shortly thereafter, the National Center for Health Statistics. (Hanlon and Pickett, 1984)

Federal programs supporting individual health services and state programs also continued to grow, both in number of health problems and types of citizens addressed. The Social Security Act was passed in 1935. One title of the act established a federal grant-in-aid program to the states for establishing and maintaining public health services and for training public health personnel. Another title increased the responsibilities of the Children's Bureau in maternal and child health and capabilities of state maternal and child health programs. The National Mental Health Act, establishing the National Institute of Mental Health as a part of NIH, was passed in 1946. This institute was also authorized to finance training programs for mental health professionals and to finance development of community mental health services in local areas, as well as to conduct and support research. The Medicare and Medicaid programs, titles 18 and 19 of the Social Security Act, were passed in 1966. These programs enabled federal payment for health services to the elderly and federal–state programs for payment for health services to the poor. (Hanlon and Pickett, 1984) The Partnership in Health Act of 1966 established a "block grant" approach for a variety of programs, providing federal funding of state and county activities in general health, tuberculosis control, dental health, home health, and mental health, among others. The block grant was used by the federal government as incentive to states and counties for further development of their health services. (Omenn, 1982) The Comprehensive Health Planning Act, passed in 1967, established a nationwide system of health planning agencies and allowed development of community health centers across the country. (Hanlon and Pickett, 1984)

State and Local Activities

Expansion of state activities in health paralleled the growth in federal activities. Many of the changes on the federal level stimulated or supported state programs. States expanded their activities in health to accommodate Medicaid, health promotion and education, and health planning, as well as many other federally sponsored programs. Medicare and Medicaid in particular had a tremendous impact at the state level. To participate in Medicaid, states had to designate a single state agency to direct the program, setting up a dichotomy between public health services and Medicaid services. Also, most states experienced a sudden growth in programs and program costs with the advent of Medicare and Medicaid. For example, federal funding for the institutionalized mentally ill became available for the first time through Medicaid, allowing expansion of these services and their costs in many states. (Turner, 1977)

Some federal programs of the 1960s also inspired growth of health services in local health departments and in private health organizations. Maternal and child health, family planning, immunization, venereal disease control, and tuberculosis control offered financial and technical assistance to local health departments to provide these services. Other federal programs developed at this time allowed funds and technical assistance to be provided directly to private health care providers, bypassing state and local government authorities. The Comprehensive Health Planning Act was an example of this trend. It allowed federal funding of neighborhood or community health centers, which were governed by boards composed of a consumer majority and related directly to the federal government for policy and program direction and finances. The National Health Service Corps Program, in which the federal government directly assigned physicians to provide medical care to citizens in underserved areas, is another example of unilateral federal action for health care.

THE LATE TWENTIETH CENTURY: A CRISIS IN CARE AND FINANCING

By the 1970s, the financial impact of the expansion in public health activities of the 1930s through the 1960s, including new public roles in the financing of medical care, began to be apparent. Per capita health expenditures increased from $198 in 1965 to $334 in 1970. During the same period, the public sector share of this sum rose from 25 percent to 37 percent. (Anderson, 1985) The social values of earlier decades came under criticism. Containing health costs became a national objective. The Health Maintenance Act of 1973, promoting health maintenance organizations as a less costly means of health care, and the National Health Planning and Resources Development Act of 1974, setting up a certification system for new health services, are examples of this effort. (Turner, 1977)

In the current decade, efforts toward cost containment continue. Although health needs and health services have not diminished, political and social values of the time encourage fiscal constraint. Current values also emphasize state responsibility for most health and welfare programs. Block grants were implemented in 1981, consolidating the federal grants-in-aid to the states into four major groups and cutting back the amount of grant money (some of the cuts were restored in 1983). Medicaid was altered to give greater leeway to the states in the design and implementation of the program, although the federal share of Medicaid financing was not changed. Changes also have been made in Medicare payment policies to restrain the increase in costs, especially for hospital care. (Omenn, 1982) At the same time, new health problems have continued to surface. AIDS, a previously unknown contagious disease, is reaching epidemic proportions. Greater numbers of hazardous by-products of industry are being produced and disposed of in the environment. Many other issues are of growing concern—asbestos exposure, side effects from pertussis vaccines, Alzheimer's disease, alcoholism and drug abuse, and homelessness are just a few. New health problems continue to be identified, conflicting with concerns about the growth of government and government spending in health.

CONCLUSION

Although science provided a foundation for public health, social values have shaped the system. The task of the public health agency has been not only to define objectives for the health care system based on facts about illness and health, but also to find means to implement health goals within a social structure. "The boundaries of public health [have changed] over time with the perception of new health and social problems and with political, economic, and ideological shifts within the government and the nation." (Fee, 1987) The history of public health has been one of identifying health problems, developing knowledge and expertise to solve problems, and rallying political and social support around the solutions.

Despite the huge successes brought about by scientific discovery and social reforms, and despite a phenomenal growth of government activities in health, the solving of public health problems has not taken place without controversy. Repeatedly, the role of the government in regulating individual behavior has been challenged. For example, as early as 1853, Britain's Board of Health was disbanded because Chadwick, its director, "claimed a wide scope for state intervention in an age when laissez-faire was the doctrine of the day." (Chave, 1984) The relationship between public health and private medical practice has also been much debated. In 1920, the New York Medical Society vehemently opposed and succeeded in defeating a proposal for a system of public rural clinics throughout the state. (Starr, 1982) Arguments about the scope of public health and the extent of public sector responsibility for health continue to this day.

The development of a scientific base for public health allowed some consistency in the public health system across the country. All of the states in the United States are involved in some manner in sanitation, laboratory investigation, collecting vital statistics, regulation of the environment, epidemiology, administering vaccines, maternal and child health, mental health, and care of the poor. How local systems conduct these programs differs greatly from area to area. Changing values over both time and place have allowed great variety in the implementation of public health programs across the country.

The following chapter, which summarizes the current public health system in the United States and public health activities in six states visited by the committee, illustrates the variety of approaches to public health which have evolved throughout the current system.

REFERENCES

Anderson, O. W. 1985. *Health Services in the United States: A Growth Enterprise Since 1875.* Health Administration Press, Ann Arbor, Mich.

Blake, Nelson M. 1956. *Water for the Cities: A History of the Urban Water Supply Problem in the United States.* Syracuse University Press, Syracuse, N.Y.

Brandt, Allan M. 1985. *No Magic Bullet: A Social History of Venereal Disease in the United States Since 1880.* Oxford University Press, New York.

Bremner, Robert H., ed. 1971. *Children and Youth in America: A Documentary History.* Harvard University Press, Cambridge, Mass.

Chave, S. P. W. 1984. "The Origins and Development of Public Health." In *Oxford Textbook of Public Health, Vol. 1: History, Determinants, Scope, and Strategies,* W. W. Holland, R. Detels, and G. Knox, eds. Oxford Medical Publications, Oxford University Press, New York.

Fee, Elizabeth. 1987. *Disease and Discovery: A History of the Johns Hopkins School of Hygiene and Public Health 1916–1939.* Johns Hopkins University Press, Baltimore.

Foley, Henry A., and Steven S. Sharfstein. 1983. *Madness and Government: Who Cares for the Mentally Ill?* American Psychiatric Press, Inc., Washington, D.C.

Goudsblom, Johan. 1986. "Public Health and the Civilizing Process." *The Milbank Quarterly* 64(2):161–88.

Grob, Gerald N. 1966. *The State and the Mentally Ill: A History of Worcester State Hospital in Massachusetts, 1830–1920.* University of North Carolina Press, Chapel Hill, N.C.

Hanlon, G., and J. Pickett. 1984. *Public Health Administration and Practice.* Times Mirror/ Mosby.

Omenn, G. S. 1982. "What's Behind Those Block Grants in Health? *New England Journal of Medicine* 306(17):1057–60.

Rosenberg, Charles E. 1962. *The Cholera Years.* University of Chicago Press, Chicago, Ill.

Rosenkrantz, Barbara G. 1972. *Public Health and the State.* Harvard University Press, Cambridge, Mass.

Rosenkrantz, Barbara G. 1974. "Cart Before the Horse: Theory, Practice, and Professional Image in American Public Health." *Journal of History of Medicine and Allied Sciences* 29:55–73

Starr, P. 1982. *The Social Transformation of American Medicine.* Basic Books, Inc., New York.

Turner, John B., editor in chief. 1977. *Encyclopedia of Social Work,* seventeenth edition. National Association of Social Workers, Washington, D.C.

Winslow, C. E. A. 1923. *The Evolution and Significance of the Modern Public Health Campaign.* Journal of Public Health Policy, South Burlington, Vt.

Wohl, Anthony S. 1983. *Endangered Lives: Public Health in Victorian Britain.* Harvard University Press, Cambridge, Mass.

4

An Assessment of the Current Public Health System: A Shattered Vision

The following chapter describes the current state of public health as observed by the committee during the course of its study. The committee viewed public health on a broad scale, considering the participation of all of the groups described in Chapter 2 which fulfill the mission of public health: government and government agencies, private providers, and voluntary organizations. This broad level is termed the *public health system**** by the committee. Within this group, the committee focused on the role and activities of the *public health agencies,* the government entities that focus the mission of public health. Other participants were considered primarily in relation to the public health agencies.

Within the United States, the role of public health agencies and their relationships with other participants in the system vary tremendously. These variations reflect tremendous differences in the fundamental concept of the definition and mission of public health across the country.

"Public health" in the United States is defined not only by the scope of health problems and their interventions in each area, but also by the values

---

* In the United States, government responsibility to protect the public's health is represented by *public health agencies,* state and local health departments, and by the federal Department of Health and Human Services. The *public health system* in the United States includes a wide array of other public agencies, such as environmental, occupational safety, mental health, developmental disability, and social service agencies at national, state, and local levels. It also includes national, state, and local private organizations and providers, such as health professional associations, citizen advocacy groups, the media, community health centers, and research foundations. Together, these participants in the system fulfill the mission of public health. The public health agencies, as the governmental representative of public health, focus this mission.

Americans have about the importance of a particular problem and the necessity of addressing that problem with public activities. The current public health system is shaped by its goals, by the health problems to be solved, and by the political system within which it functions.

Because public health problems are often addressed on a state and local rather than a national scale, goals are set within different political systems. Different communities have different health problems and they have appreciably different political and social organizations and values. So, public health systems in these communities vary widely and offer widely differing public health services.

Viewed from a national perspective, the national public health system is a scene of tremendous variety and disarray as different communities work out different solutions to public health problems.

This chapter describes how the committee conducted its study of the national public health system and then describes the committee's observations of the system in specific areas it visited. Anecdotes from local areas are used as representative data, reflecting trends observed on a national level from published data, literature, and committee experience. Major characteristics of the entire system are briefly summarized in this chapter. A more detailed description of the public health system can be found in Appendix A to this report.

VIEWING THE SYSTEM

For this study, the committee decided that its conclusions about the current public health system would benefit from firsthand observation that could augment analysis of more inclusive information summarized in this chapter and in Appendix A. Therefore, it made site visits to the state capitals and several local areas in California, Mississippi, New Jersey, South Dakota, Washington, and West Virginia. In each state committee members and staff spoke with hundreds of citizens who work in and are served by the public health system. The committee also held four open meetings in Las Vegas, Boston, New Orleans, and Chicago at which several hundred citizens and public health practitioners spoke.

The committee realized that not all variations in the country could possibly be examined in site visits. However, the committee felt that a careful selection of sites in six states would present sufficient variety to illustrate the range of health problems and public health activities that exist across the nation. The areas visited within the states were chosen to reflect a variety of geographical locations, urban–rural mix, health problems, population mix and economic status, public health agency organization, and array of public health services. (See Appendix D for a fuller description of the selection process and the plan for the site visits.) Individual sites were treated as illustrative rather than representative of public health practice in the United States or as exhaustive case studies. But the committee believes that these illustrations illuminate fundamental issues for the entire system.

Among the six states, population density ranged from one of the most densely populated states to one of the least. In one, the proportion of urban dwellers was 16 percent; in another, 95 percent. Per capita personal income in the states ranged from $8,857 to $15,182. Percentage of high school graduates in the state varied from 55 percent to 77 percent, and unemployment from 6.2 percent to 13 percent. The states had different percentages of minority groups, including blacks, Hispanics, Asians, and Native Americans, as well as populations of illegal immigrants. State and local health expenditures per person were as low as $72, and as high as $172. Physicians per 100,000 population ranged from 107 to 230. (U.S. Department of Commerce, 1986) In some states, private health resources and services were abundant, and in some they were very scarce. Some state governments put a great deal of emphasis on carrying out the public health mission, and some put very little emphasis on it.

At each site, committee members and committee staff spoke with state and local health officers; state and local health department directors and program administrators; state and local environmental, social service, and mental health agency personnel; representatives of local and state government; representatives of hospital, medical, and nursing professional associations and of citizen organizations; health professionals; administrators and board members in private and public hospitals and clinics; journalists; and professors of medicine and of public health. The committee conducted a total of more than 350 interviews.

Interviews focused mainly on health problems identified by those interviewed and the means by which the system was successfully or unsuccessfully handling these problems. Identified problems included teenage pregnancy, medical care for indigent populations, safe water supply, the disposal of hazardous materials, AIDS, alcoholism, mental health, prenatal care, smoking prevention, access to medical care, sexually transmitted diseases, infant mortality, home health, long-term care, Alzheimer's disease, injuries, malpractice, childhood vaccines, substance abuse, asbestos, radiation control, and dental health. Many views of public health were expressed, ranging from "it affects everybody" to "it's whatever the market won't do." Descriptions of public health agencies varied from "the public health department is the champion/guardian of the public's health" to "I don't know what they do" and "public health professionals are 'also rans' in the medical profession."

Federal health officials were also interviewed during the study. And a subgroup of the committee made a visit to Toronto, Canada, to discuss the Canadian public health system with several health officials and health professionals.

Of the four meetings to which members of the public were invited, the first was held during the annual meeting of the American Public Health Association in Las Vegas, Nevada, in September 1986. The other meetings were held in Boston, Massachusetts, in October 1986; New Orleans, Louisiana, February 1987; and Chicago, Illinois, May 1987. More than 350 people, including citizens of 39 states, the District of Columbia, and Canada, attended these meetings. Attendees included state health commissioners and state health agency officials; local health officers; deans and professors of medical schools, schools of public health, nursing schools, and schools of public administration; federal health officials; consumer representatives; physicians, nurses, social workers, health educators, and mental health professionals; representatives of state medical associations, state nurse's associations, and state social worker's associations; directors of public hospitals and community health centers; members of state boards of health; and representatives from nonprofit associations. Topics discussed at these meetings included the philosophy and scope of public health, specific issues in public health organization, management, leadership and resources, and particular health needs.

The committee also held a special meeting on education and training for public health. It was attended by deans and professors from all of the schools of public health, representatives of other educational programs providing public health training, state and local government officials, representatives from national organizations focused on health education, and state and local public health professionals from the field. Presentations were given and discussions held on a variety of issues pertaining to education and practice, including the nature of professional education, the nature of public health as a profession, the relationship between public health practice and education, and the role and activities of schools of public health in educating health professionals. The proceedings of this meeting will be published by the Institute of Medicine in a separate volume.

Additionally, the committee collected and reviewed extensive amounts of current and historical literature and data on public health problems and the public health system.

Although the committee looked into a broad array of issues in public health, it concentrated on those problems of a public scope rather than health services aimed primarily at the individual. In some cases, this distinction was not easy to make. For instance, most mental health services are directed toward the individual, but all states sponsor mental health programs. Rather than attempt to study both fields, or study such a vast and important topic in an adjunct manner, the committee decided to focus on those aspects of mental health that substantially overlap with public health. During its study, the committee spoke with a number of mental health professionals; discussed several mental health problems that are dealt with on a public level, including alcoholism, substance abuse, Alzheimer's disease, and homelessness; and discussed the role of public health in coordinating with mental health programs. But the committee did not make a separate study of the provision of mental health services to individuals, a very large public responsibility in all states. Likewise, the committee's approach to social and human services, many of which intersect with public health concerns, was limited to those having direct interaction with public health activities.

The committee paid principal attention to public health at the state and local levels. An extensive amount of information was collected from the federal government, but the federal role in public health was mostly considered as it relates to state and local health systems.

THE PUBLIC HEALTH SYSTEM

This section describes the public health system as observed by the committee in its research. The discussion focuses on state and local public health agencies—the central agents in the public health system—and their activities and describes other components of the system in relation to health agencies.

A brief summary of the organization and scope of the public health system activities at the national, state, and local levels is followed by a description of the ways the system operates in the specific localities visited by the committee in the summer of 1986. Observations on issues and problems of the public health system are drawn primarily from the site visits conducted by the committee, but information presented in meetings and literature and data collected by the committee are also taken into account.

SUMMARY OF THE NATIONAL PUBLIC HEALTH SYSTEM

State

The U.S. Constitution empowers state governments to protect the health and welfare of their citizens through the exercise of police power. States have thus become the central authorities in the nation's public health system. (Grad, 1981)

Each of the 54 states and territories of the United States has designated an agency for public health. The organization and leadership of these agencies vary. Some are parts of state superagencies for human services, and some are independent. Some are combined with mental health or environmental agencies, and some are not. (Public Health Foundation, 1986) Some state health agency directors are required to be physicians with public health experience, and some are administrators with management experience. (American Medical Association, 1984)

The state public health agencies carry out each of the public health functions described in Chapter 2: assessment, policy development, and assurance of access to health services. Although general functions are the same, scope of activities and specific activities of health agencies vary tremendously. Some states conduct a wide array of services, and some only a few. Some concentrate on assessment and policy development activities, some concentrate almost solely on assuring access and delivering personal health services. State resources designated to health also vary. (Public Health Foundation, 1986)

Finally, state public health agencies differ in their relationships with other state agencies involved in health, in their relationships with local health authorities, and in their relationships with the private sector. Some work closely together, some rarely communicate, and some openly compete.

A more detailed description of state health agencies and their leadership, organization, activities, and resources is presented in Appendix A.

Local

Local health agencies are the critical components of the public health system that directly deliver public health services to citizens. Local governments and local agencies are invested with power by their state governments. (Grad, 1981) Although local authorities may carry out each of the public health functions outlined in Chapter 2, they are generally substantially more involved in assurance activities, largely the actual provision of services to the population. (Miller and Moos, 1981; Public Health Foundation, 1986)

Differences in geography and systems of government allow local health agencies to vary even more greatly than state agencies. Some local health agencies are municipal, some serve a county, and some serve groups of counties, or districts. (Miller and Moos, 1981) Some are directed by full-time physician health officers with public health experience; some are run by part-time administrators with little public health experience. (Miller et al., 1977) Some local areas have large, sophisticated health departments that carry out all public health functions with little dependence on the state. Many areas have smaller, more limited health departments that work in conjunction with, or as a branch of, the state health department. And some local areas have no public health department at all. (Public Health Foundation, 1986) Local health agencies also vary considerably in their procurement and allocation of resources.

Finally, local health agencies vary in their relationships with other local agencies and with private providers. Some are components of local super-agencies; some are independent. Many rely on private providers to augment services; some have little to do with private providers.

Local health agencies and their activities are also summarized in Appendix A to this report.

Federal

The federal government plays a strong role in public health. The federal government conducts public health activities through its power to regulate interstate commerce and its power to tax and spend for the public welfare. (Grad, 1981)

The Public Health Service of the Department of Health and Human Services is the main federal authority in health. The federal government is involved in each of the public health functions described in Chapter 2, but its main efforts are in assessment, research, and policy and program development. Most of its assurance activities are conducted through funding contracts with states, local areas, and providers, who actually carry out the service. Some assurance activities are directly carried out by the federal government. (Hanlon and Pickett, 1984)

Federal activities in health are described further in Appendix A.

Resources

In 1984, the nation spent about $387 billion on health care. This figure includes both government and private expenditures for public health programs and personal medical care. Public only, including federal, state, and local government spending, totaled about $160 billion. (Bureau of Data Management and Strategy, Health Care Financing Administration, 1985) Federal spending alone (including Medicare and Medicaid) was about $112 billion or about $460 per person. (U.S. Department of Commerce, 1986) State spending, (excluding Medicaid) totaled about $6 billion, averaging $23 to $26 per person. (Public Health Foundation, 1986; U.S. Department of Commerce, 1986) Local government spending totaled about $2.5 billion. (Public Health Foundation, 1986)

In all levels of government, spending on personal health services greatly outweighed spending on population-based public health functions. For example, the health portion of the budget of the Health and Human Services Department included $95 billion to finance the Medicare and Medicaid programs. The budget for the U.S. Public Health Service, including the Centers for Disease Control; the National Institutes of Health; the Health Resources and Services Administration; and the Alcohol Abuse, Drug Abuse, and Mental Health Administration, totaled only $10 billion. (Executive Office of the President, Office of Management and Budget, 1987) State health agencies spent nearly 75 percent of their funds on personal health services, about $4 billion, while spending less than 1 percent on planning activities, about 3 percent on laboratory analysis and research, and about 9 percent on all resources development. Local health agencies spent, on the average, about 58 percent of their funds on personal health services. (Public Health Foundation, 1986)

National and public spending on health care has been a subject of great controversy in the 1980s. Public spending on health care increased dramatically throughout the 1960s and 1970s. Much of the federal and state increases reflect increases in spending on personal health services and medical care. The Medicare and Medicaid programs were initiated in 1966. While aggregate state health agency spending increased at about 4 percent annually between 1976 and 1984, the proportion of their finances spent on personal health services increased from 48 to 58 percent. (Public Health Foundation, 1987) Spending on assessment and policy activities has not increased so dramatically.

In the 1980s, cutbacks in public spending for health care became a national goal. In 1981, federal block grants were initiated which consolidated numerous federal health programs into two blocks. These block grants included a 25 percent cut in funding to states for their programs. (Omenn, 1982) Since 1981, these funds have been partially restored. From 1984 to 1985, the maternal and child health block grant increased 16 percent, while the preventive services block grant increased 21 percent. (Public Health Foundation, 1986, 1987) The GNP growth factor for this period was at 6.8 percent. (U.S. Department of Commerce, 1986) At the same time, state health agency spending increased about 10 percent. (Public Health Foundation, 1986, 1987) Nonetheless, these increases are modest compared to increases in some other social programs. During the same period, funding for drug enforcement programs, a particular social goal for this period, increased 550 percent. (Executive Office of the President, Office of Management and Budget, 1987)

Increases in public health spending are not keeping pace with the growing need for assessment, policy development, and assurance activities demanded by the range of immediate and impending crises and ongoing problems in public health as discussed in Chapter 1, particularly in the assessment and policy development areas. Additionally, resources for particular needs to fulfill the mission of public health, such as leadership training, are being cut back. Federal funding for health professions training is being phased out, and state resources for leadership training and encouraging health leaders to take public positions are limited. (Council of State Governments, 1985; Executive Office of the President, Office of Management and Budget, 1987)

Federal, state, and local resources for health are discussed more fully in Appendix A.

Other Actors

Additionally, it should be noted that other government agencies, such as federal, state, and local agencies in mental health, environmental health, and social services, have an impact on the public health system. And private entities, such as health professional organizations, citizen activist groups, health care providers, and voluntary health organizations, also play a crucial role. These other components of the public health system are briefly discussed in Appendix A.

THE PUBLIC HEALTH SYSTEM AS OBSERVED BY THE COMMITTEE

In the six states visited by the committee, six different public health systems were observed. The states varied in their concept of and in the importance they placed on public health. The health agencies in each state varied in organization, authority, activities, and resources. The other actors in the system differed in their participation in public health issues and in their relationships with the health agencies. Nonetheless, many common themes emerged between the sites. The need for more authoritative leadership and greater flexibility in public health was often voiced. Also coveted were organization, consistent services, and the capacity to maintain staff, finances, and information. And particular functions of public health and programs of health agencies were seen as fundamental by many persons interviewed.

The following section describes characteristics of the six areas visited by the committee and discusses problems and successes of the health systems in these areas as told by their participants.

Organization of Health Agencies

Among the six states, two state health agencies were divisions of super-agencies. One state health agency was also the mental health authority; two were also the state Medicaid agency. Five were organized into functional divisions, and one by service populations. The organizational relationships between the state and local health agencies ranged from one in which all local health agencies were largely independent to one in which all local health agencies were run by the state health agency. One state had 114 local health agencies; one had only one.

The local health agencies also differed. In one of the states, local health agencies were predominantly municipal; in the rest of the states, they were predominantly or entirely county. Two states had both municipal and county health departments. Two local agencies were large and had numerous divisions and hundreds of staff; the rest were small, had only a few programs, and a dozen or two staff at most. In one of the states visited, most of the local areas had no health department at all, but had a private physician who served as a local health officer. Participants of public meetings described other states in which some local areas have no health department. In these areas, there are almost no locally based public health programs.

Variation in organization of health agencies existed not only between states but within states. For example, in two cases a superagency existed at one level but not at the other; in several, services that were not combined at one level were combined at the other. For example, in one state the state health agency was part of a superagency combined with social services, but separate from mental health and environmental services. The local health agency visited in this state was independent from the social services agency but had mental health and environmental divisions.

Organization of state and local agencies also changed over time. Several of the health departments visited had been organized several different ways throughout their histories. In one state, the state health agency had been completely reorganized a few weeks before the committee's visit. In another state, the section of the health agency dealing with AIDS had recently moved up three levels in the hierarchy and was growing 10-fold in staff and finances. In another, the number of local health agencies had recently been reduced by half, from more than 200 to 114. This had been done mostly by combining small local health agencies. In another state, many programs started by the health department had been relocated to other agencies.

The state of flux in health agencies is due partly to the difficulty of segregating health-related functions. For example, there was much sharing of and confusion over environmental responsibilities. The state of flux is also due to the changing circumstances with which health agencies must deal. As new problems such as AIDS and toxics develop, new programs are set up for dealing with them. Or problems become of increased social and political concern, and new programs are developed or existing ones are given increased importance.

The different patterns of organization in the six states illustrated how the states dealt with the main difficulty in arranging a public health agency, namely, coordinating an extensive array of different types of services that relate to other agencies. One state handled this problem with a health and social services agency and a separate environmental agency. Health programs that addressed needs of a particular population were grouped with social service programs in different divisions of the health and social services agency. Assessment and education activities were dispersed throughout these programs. At the local level, both health and social services agencies existed. In another state, health and social services programs were kept separate, but health and environmental services were combined at both the state and local levels. In a third state, the health agency, the social service agency, and the environmental agency were all separate. Some local health departments were independent, and some were parts of health and social service agencies. Environmental services were handled by multicounty commissions.

The various arrangements in the states illustrated problems with combining services and problems with separating them. In the state with the superagency, local health officials and some others felt that public health initiatives were lost in the superagency. Some of the state public health officials even expressed a desire to be grouped 'with the environmental agency, as they felt this would be a more visible location. In a state where the Medicaid program and the health agency were separate, Medicaid policies about financing various health services were set without health agency input. Yet in another state in which the programs were grouped, Medicaid policy seemed to dominate health policy.

The committee found that, regardless of organization, health services were often fragmented along organizational lines. In one state, substance abuse programs were handled by the state health agency, but mental health services were the responsibility of the social services agency. Almost no communication took place between the programs. In this same state, the health agency and the environmental agency were also separate, but inspections and data collection activities of both agencies were coordinated at the local level. In another state, local health agencies were responsible for environmental health, but not hazardous waste disposal. When accidents occurred in transport of hazardous waste, health authorities were called at the last moment to inspect the site. In the meantime, they had no knowledge of the potential dangers of the situation. Participants in each of the open meetings described the fragmentation that occurs among social, mental health, and public health services when they are not coordinated.

Leadership

Five of the states required that the state health officer be a physician; one did not. In five of the states, all of the local health officers were physicians. In one, most were nurses or sanitarians. In many agencies, the health officer directs the agency. But in others, the health officer and the director hold different positions in the agency. In three states and in all but one of the local areas visited, the health officer was the director of the agency. In three states and in one local area the health officer reported to an administrative director. In two largely rural states, private physicians served part-time as local health officers who worked with the local agency when there was one.

The variety of requirements and arrangements for health agency leaders provided examples of strengths and weaknesses in public health leadership. In one state, the health officer was a physician, was director of the state agency, had authority over all local services, and reported to a state board of health. In another state, the health officer, also a physician, filled an advisory position and had no line of authority. The administrator of the agency seldom called on this health officer for advice. Local health officers in the first state were physicians, were state employees, and had jurisdiction over multicounty areas. Local health officers in the second were private physicians with few appointed responsibilities. As one local health officer in this state put it, "Being a health officer is not a big thing these days."

Strength of state and local leadership also differed within states. In the state in which the state health officer had little authority and local health officers had few responsibilities, several examples of strong local leadership were found. In another state, the state health officer was a physician who reported directly to the governor and was well respected, but the local health officer was seen by many as lacking initiative.

Several aspects of health agency leadership were observed. The first was a trend toward more directors of health agencies with backgrounds in general administration. In two of the states, the health officers were former directors of the health agency and had been repositioned to report to an administrator heading the agency. Another aspect was an association between the number of political appointees in a state health agency and health agency consciousness of gubernatorial or legislative priorities. In one state, four tiers of health agency directors were political appointees, and the agency was very responsive to the legislature. Another state health department was described as "very close to the governor." The third aspect was rapid turnover in health agency leadership. In three of the states and one local area, the health officer had been on the job less than a year. Several health agency administrators were equally new. One state had had three different state health officers in 5 years. Instability of leadership was often mentioned as a problem. One observer said, "The health department has a zillion problems—a different director every year." Some health officers, however, had been in their positions for dozens of years.

The committee noted that several leaders of health agencies in the states were praised by elected officials and health leaders in the private sector for their determination, their ability to solve health problems, and their ability to work with others. One state agency was credited with drastically reducing the infant mortality rate in the state by providing maternity services, family planning services, and child health services to poor citizens. The state's infant mortality rate had dropped from 18.7 in 1980 to 14.4 in 1984. In another state, a local agency was praised for its handling of AIDS programs in cooperation with local hospitals and community groups. The agency was working with a community group seeking to coordinate community-based services, providing acute services at a county public hospital, and seeking establishment of a hospice program.

However, the committee found that the majority of agencies were criticized for their lack of leadership. Those outside the health agency said that they should be able to look to the health agency for direction on health issues, but couldn't. One said, "There isn't any policy, the health department should take the lead." Those inside the agency said they should be more forward thinking. "You need to get information and then make a decision, not sit back and see which way the wind is blowing." These views were also brought out at open meetings.

Several factors contribute to the poor image of public health leadership in many communities. In some states, overall public and political interest in public health was low, and the ability of public health agencies to act as leaders suffered from this disinterest. One of the states that was facing severe economic problems had few resources dedicated to health, a small state health agency, and limited services. Yet many citizens supported this minimalist orientation to health, both for financial reasons and because they believe in limited government. Said one citizen representative, "Our state doesn't have a tradition of helping. It's not a rich state." And from the same state, "This state was big on privatization long before Reagan." In another state, public health was characterized as lacking political attractiveness. Said one state health official, "Supervisors don't generally give money to health—they're into building roads." And a nurse–legislator in a third state said that the legislature allocated $3 million to renovate highway bathrooms, but only $1 million for prenatal care.

Public health agencies also suffered from the generally poor image of bureaucrats. A characteristic comment was, "Public health people are lousy administrators, out of touch, encapsulated in their public health world." A state legislator exclaimed of public health officials, "They're eunuchs! They're consummate bureaucrats!" Public health workers were described by many in the medical community as passive survivors, "also rans" in the world of health. Even people within the public health system made negative comments about agency leadership. A local health agency official criticized the state agency, "Some of us are frustrated by a sit-on-your-hands health department." Yet many public health workers expressed satisfaction with their jobs.

The image of public health agencies also suffers because the job is a difficult one. Health agencies deal with numerous critical issues at the same time and often have few resources to respond to new issues and little political authority to rally support. The most frequent perception of the health department by legislators and citizens was of a slow and inflexible bureaucracy battling with chaos, fighting to meet crises, and behaving in an essentially reactive manner. In more than one of the states, this appeared to be close to the truth. One state health official revealed, "Just getting through the day is the only real objective of the senior administrator." Even people who praised health departments often did so in a qualified way, mentioning lack of resources or lack of attention paid to public health accomplishments. A typical comment was made by the director of a state hospital association:

"The hospitals respect the local health departments, but they believe that there is no way they can do the job because they are underfunded and understaffed."

Lack of adequate compensation for the leaders charged with these difficult responsibilities makes recruitment and retention of able leaders more problematic in many states. In 1986, 22 states paid their chief health official less than $60,000 per annum. Of these states, 7 paid less than $45,000. Only 5 states paid this important official more than $80,000 (see Appendix A for a full listing of these salaries). (Council of State Governments, 1987)

Health agencies also suffer from lack of visibility. "The public visibility of the state health service is nil," was a frequent sentiment. Some of the health agency's low profile is due to its successes. A lot of public health activities, such as sanitation, are considered routine and are taken for granted by the community. One local citizen said, "The public is unaware of the county health department. They do a good job, so people forget about them." Additionally, much of the goal of public health is to stop hazardous situations from arising. A public health professor pointed out, "You don't get grateful patients for preventing problems." To combat this problem, some agencies maintained a close relationship with the media, using the press to gain public attention to issues. One local health agency frequently contacted the health affairs reporter at the local paper. But most were mistrustful of the press, and saw it used more as a tool against them. Some departments felt that the press was used by others to draw attention to issues and force the department to act.

Despite the difficulties, some state and local departments were praised for their motivation, for their responsiveness to a particular health issue, for innovations in working with private providers and the community. The committee was genuinely impressed with the high level of dedication it observed throughout the system. Given the tremendous difficulties in some areas—a coal mining county in which one-third of the workforce was idle; a county with a flow of indigent refugees coming across the border in need of local resources; cities with large populations of homeless citizens, including many young adults and many substance abusers; and large numbers of farm failures in a rural county—the committee found it admirable that the agencies addressed as many health issues as they did.

Some criticisms of health agencies are not deserved. But the difficulties in leadership and the overall poor image of public health exposed in the interviews cannot be ignored. Many state and local health officers felt thwarted by the political system and numerous conflicting demands. But the legislators, county supervisors, and citizenry in all but a few locations felt that the health officers were often unresponsive to the needs and desires of the broader society.

Range of Activities

The activities carried out by the six states and local areas visited by the committee differed along the many lines already mentioned. The range of services in each state is shown in Table 4.1. All of the state agencies were involved in assessment, policymaking, and assurance of access to educational, environmental, and personal health services. The two largest local health agencies also conducted activities in each function. The other local health agencies concentrated mostly on assuring access to health services and providing health services, particularly environmental and personal services. The extent of any one state or local agency's involvement in a function differed depending on the health issues in the area, the perception of need for a particular service, community priorities, and availability of resources.

Activities were also carried out through a variety of arrangements between state and local agencies and between public and private providers. One state and the local areas within it spent a majority of effort on directly providing personal health services. Another state focused its efforts on inspections and environmental regulation. Nearly all personal health care was delivered by the private sector and three public hospitals. One state agency spent most of its effort on assessment and policy development, while the local areas within the state concentrated on educational, environmental, and personal services. Another agency handled assessment activities and environmental inspections, but left it up to the private sector to carry out local educational and personal health services. In some cases, the health agency was less involved in an activity, but the function was fulfilled by other agencies or by the private sector. And in some cases, the health agency was less involved, and the function was not taken over by others.

Assessment

All of the state and local agencies were involved in some data collection, epidemiology, screening for health problems, and laboratory analysis. Even a state with few resources dedicated to health conducted all of these activities. The only source of variation in assessment activities lay in the extent of the state or local agency's involvement. For example, four states had state centers for vital statistics. Two collected statistics, but had no separate centers. Two of the states provided screening for a large variety of disorders, including communicable and chronic disease, genetic disorders, developmental disabilities, hearing, vision, hypertension, anemia, tuberculosis, and sexually transmitted diseases. The other four screened for only a few diseases and disorders. One of these concentrated almost wholly on hypertension and sexually transmitted disease. (Public Health Foundation, 1986) All of the states had laboratories, but only two of the local areas had their own

TABLE 4.1   Activities of Six State Agencies, 1984[a]

	Number of States ($n = 6$)		Number of States ($n = 6$)
I. ASSESSMENT		III. ASSURANCE (*continued*)	
A. Data Collection		A. Inspection (*continued*)	
Vital Records	6	Housing, Public, Lodging, Recreational Facility Safety	6
Mobidity	3		
Health Facilities	4		
Health Manpower	5		
Health System Funds	5	Health Facility Safety	5
Health Interview Surveys	2	B. Licensing	5
Health Trends Analysis	3	C. Health Education Education	5
Health Status Assessment	5	Health Promotion, Disease Prevention	2
B. Epidemiology		D. Environment	
Communicable Disease	6	Air Quality	3
Health Screening	6	Occupational Health and Safety	5
Laboratory Analysis	6	Radiation Control	6
C. Research		Solid Waste Management	3
Research Projects	4	Hazardous Waste Management	3
Laboratory Research	1	Public Water Supply	5
II. POLICY DEVELOPMENT		Individual Water Supply	4
A. Policy		Sewage Disposal	5
Goals Developed Through Health Assessments	1	E. Personal Health	
Standards for Local Health Agencies	5	Maternal and Child Health	6
B. Health Planning		Home Health	4
State Health Planning	2	Immunizations	6
Categorical Plans	5	Dental Health	6
Certificate of Need	5	Mental Health	5
III. ASSURANCE		Alcohol Abuse	5
A. Inspection		Drug Abuse	5
Food and Milk Control	6	Chronic Disease	6
Product Safety, Substance Control	3	Inpatient Facilities	2
		F. Resources Development	6

[a]This list is a representative subset of activities listed for all states in Tables A.4 through A.6 of Appendix A.

SOURCE: Public Health Foundation, 1986, pp. 2, 3, 10, 19, 27, 33, 37, 38, 39, 40, 41.

laboratories. The remaining local areas relied on state or private laboratories.

In addition to the collection and analysis of the types of data listed in Table 4.1, most of the states mentioned seeking information on specific health problems as they became of interest. In several states, the number of teen pregnancies was being tracked. In one, a growing number of measles cases being reported by private physicians in a local area drew local, then state attention and caused the state to increase efforts in screening and immunizing against measles. The county medical examiner's office in one area had developed a tracking and reporting system for injuries. The emergency medical system, over which the examiner had authority, was operating a surveillance system. One local health agency was testing private homes for indoor air pollution. Two state agencies were spending an extensive amount of time tracking AIDS cases. Another two state agencies were testing private water supplies for specific contaminants.

The state and local agencies were also involved collecting special information to evaluate programs. One was evaluating the effect of its prenatal care program. Another was evaluating its nutrition service. A third was monitoring the level of immunization rates. And two states were evaluating family planning services.

A few of the states and local areas were also involved in research on specific health problems. Some research projects were statewide efforts, involving state and local government, various agencies, and private providers. One state legislature had designated a commission composed of researchers, professional association members, and public and private providers to study the uninsured population in the state. This state also had a multiagency committee researching the epidemiology of radiation. Another state had a commission appointed by the governor to study Alzheimer's disease. Other projects were health-agency-initiated. For example, one state agency had a grant from a private foundation to study the psychological effects of testing and the benefits of counseling for AIDS victims.

Despite the number of special information-gathering and research projects, many participants also reported that there were health problems for which data were not being gathered. Health officials in two of the rural states described uncertainty about the health status and needs of populations in remote areas. In one state, health practitioners felt that mental health problems, stress, alcoholism, and injuries related to those conditions were being greatly underreported and greatly underestimated. Citizens in one local area were concerned about the lack of a system for diagnosing and reporting effects of environmental toxins on individuals. These citizens had suffered many health problems they believed to be related to their water supply and had sued a company with a landfill in their area. But they had had difficulty defining and proving the extent of damage because epidemiological and medical data on such problems are scarce.

Numerous other problems were mentioned concerning information and assessment activities. The most frequently mentioned problems in site visits and open meetings were difficulties in obtaining useful data and the failure to share information. Many people described the paucity of useful data on various issues, the difficulty of obtaining data, and the problems that arose from limited data. One local health officer complained, "The only vital statistics collected are those for the federal registry. We can get very little data that are actually useful." Conversely, a state health official in a different state said, "We can detect more than we can do anything about." Frequently, people in states mentioned the need to collect their own data on particular issues. Several local areas reviewed studies of problems by hospitals or universities in the area. Many mentioned receiving information or assistance from the federal Centers for Disease Control on a particular issue. People in states and localities frequently mentioned obtaining data from agencies at levels of government different from their own and from the private sector, particularly private health care providers. In many areas, gathering information is a collective effort, although in some areas, difficulties in obtaining information from other agencies or the private sector was mentioned. And sometimes a lack of uniformity among data from different sources, particularly among Medicaid, social services, and public health programs, was cited as a problem.

A second issue frequently mentioned about data was its lack of timeliness. In local areas, information is collected by the health department and private providers and passed on to the state, which passes it on to the Centers for Disease Control and other federal agencies, who analyze the data and report them back to the states and local areas. A time lapse of 2 years between collection and dissemination is common. One local health official said data had not even been collected for 2 years. Many local areas mentioned the need for increased state specific efforts and quicker turnaround time in order for data to be more useful.

State officials also described the difficulty of making data meaningful for politicians and the public. Data are gathered and used by the health department, but are also used to promote policies and initiate programs. Many health officials discussed the need to make health information understandable to decision-makers. Many also described the need to provide non-frightening, accurate information about risk to the public. One agency had been swamped by requests for information following the disaster at Chernobyl.

Some agency officials mentioned the difficulty of responding to all of the requests they receive for information. One state agency spent so much time responding to legislative requests that highly placed officials sometimes had to neglect regular responsibilities. One staff person at a local agency confided that internal requests were answered first, governmental requests second, and public requests sometimes not at all.

Finally, many health officials discussed the need to use data to prioritize programs. Data can be used both to document need and to avoid need. One state health official in a state with a large maternal and child health program said, "It's easier to justify spending money on infant mortality because you've got numbers to show need. The water supply doesn't get money because it's preventive and nobody is sick." Another person in an economically disadvantaged state said of many health problems, "We don't want to know; if we did, it would cost us money." Another state-level person described frustration with the failure to use data in policy decisions. The complaint was that "basic public health data are used effectively in making policy recommendations, but the ultimate decision is political." In another state, a state health official acknowledged they were collecting data on birth defects and cancer, but couldn't use them because "the governor wants to keep government limited."

Policy Development

All of the state agencies were involved in policy-making and planning activities, although their involvement differed. In one state, half the agency was devoted to health planning and regulation. Three of the states had special policy analysis units. In another, very little policy development and planning was done. Only one local agency, one of the largest, was involved in health policy development.

Each of the state agencies was also involved in special policy development and planning activities. Five had developed standards for local health agencies, and one of them was involved in implementing the federally initiated model standards for community preventive health services in four of its counties. The sixth state had set statewide objectives for health promotion and disease prevention based on statewide health assessments and on national objectives published in the federal *1990 Objectives for the Nation.*

Several of the states were involved in efforts to set new policies on new issues. Initiatives came from state and local government, from citizen groups, and from health agencies. In one state, legislative staff were working on legislation restricting smoking in public buildings, while the health agency staff were designing and implementing health education programs in smoking prevention and cessation. In several states, legislators and health providers were seeking new policies on providing health care for the indigent, and two states had special task forces on health care for the indigent. In one of these states, the legislature was developing, with the assistance of the local health agencies and private associations, a basic set of health services to be made available to all residents. In another, hospitals were lobbying for changes in reimbursement policy. This state health agency was also investigating the possibility of providing free needles to intravenous drug users in order to inhibit the spread of AIDS. Another state had recently adopted legislation requiring reporting of all adverse reactions to vaccines, mostly due to the efforts of one citizen's group.

States and local agencies differed in their involvement with and views of local government, the public, and the political process in helping with policy development. Some agencies would seek the support of legislators and county executives, and they would contact the press to gain publicity for new programs and policies. As one state health officer said, "Part of our job is to sell this stuff." Another state agency was regularly contacted by the state legislature for information to back legislative proposals. But in another state, most of the new policies were developed by legislative staff without the aid of the health department; the health department was viewed by the legislature as "politically infantile." One local area sometimes conducted citizen polls on new policy proposals that city government had recently had a referendum on whether health services for homeless people should be offered through the agency and had conducted a telephone survey on indigent care problems. But other health officials viewed the political process as distorting health needs and warping priorities. One state official said, "Every time we get a new governor, the leaders change, and the ideas change. Near the end of the term, they stop caring." And, from the same state, "The legislature likes public health, but we lose out on appropriations night." Others avoided involvement with the public. A health official in another state said, "When you allow people to participate, you are implicitly saying that you will take their advice, or at least listen carefully."

Many state agencies described how difficult it is to plan, to control policy, and to prioritize programs. Several participants in the system felt that planning and policy development were not done enough by their agency. Although one state agency official described the agency's use of needs assessments to justify programs, another said, "We have looked at individual problems rather than the big picture. We haven't sat down and examined relative health threats. For example, air pollution isn't hip anymore, but its still a big problem." A local official said, "We should look at issues up front, not when they hit us in the face." Many described the difficulty of balancing new needs with old issues. One state official said, "Sometimes we tend to focus on new problems and slight things that have been around for 50 years but have not been licked." In this agency, officials considered sexually transmitted diseases other than AIDS to be a continuing serious problem that received no political attention.

Some agencies said that priorities are set based on health crises, such as an environmental accident or a disease outbreak. One health official said, "Gripping stories have an impact on policy." And a legislative representative commented, "All advances in this state are built around crises." Other participants said programs are prioritized because there is public interest in an issue, or because an individual leader takes interest. From a state official, "Decisions come because political leaders perceive what the public wants. If they say do it, you resign or you do it." And, "When something scares the people who pass the laws, you get change."

It was also said that programs are arranged because money is available for them. "The categorically needy are at the top of our list, because we get federal money for them." One county administrator exclaimed, "You give us the money, and we'll implement the program!" A state agency was described as doing "only what the federal government pays for." Participants in one of the open meetings described the substantial influence federal funding has on state ability to set policies. Even though block grants gave more leeway to state agencies, the simultaneous cut in finances thwarted the ability to plan and set new policies.

Some states felt that federal assistance in setting priorities was useful, and others did not. Some were pleased that federal restrictions that had accompanied categorical grants had been lessened through block grants. One state health officer said, "Now we can do what we want instead of the feds dictating to us." A local health officer in the same state said, "The silver lining in the loss of federal funds is that now people realize they'll have to set priorities themselves, rather than wait for some planner with money to do it." But officials in another agency said, "When the president adopted new federalism, he also threw the problems back to the local level—what's happening here is that we're trying to step into a void." Some states still felt restricted by federal spending policies. One state agency official decried the state's inability to provide services for mental health and alcoholism, while spending more than justifiable on maternal and child health. Another complained that unexpected surpluses in the Medicaid program "get plowed into pork barrels at the last minute."

Some agencies mentioned using the federal *1990 Objectives for the Nation* for setting new objectives, standards, and priorities. One state was using these objectives to support a new orientation toward health promotion. Two used them as a basis for a statewide health status analysis, upon which they intended to base new policies. But the director of the health promotion programs in one state complained, "The 1990 Objectives and Model Standards—how do you prioritize them? They don't tell you which issues are more important." Federal standards for resource allocation were also discussed. In rural areas, these standards are particularly difficult to maintain. One local hospital board member said, "If we have to adhere to national standards, we'll have to close our ICU, and the next one is 50 miles away." A local health officer stated, "A small rural hospital is an anachronism until you consider geography. In trying to maintain services in a sparsely populated area, you don't practice any one thing too much. Does that make a compromise in quality of care, or do you force people to travel?"

A few of the state agencies also mentioned restrictive state policies. In one state, legislative approval was required for all program expenditures, item by item. In another, legislative approval was required for all agency regulations. And local areas occasionally discussed difficulties with state policies. One local official said, "County health departments do what we're told to do— programs are either federal or state, and there's little leeway to do what you want."

Assurance of Health Services

All of the six states were involved in regulating and licensing health facilities and programs and conducting inspections. One state agency devoted half its efforts to planning and regulatory activities. Another limited its regulatory activities to licensing and inspecting health facilities and recreational facilities.

Health services provided by the six states and localities covered a broad range of health needs. The sites had many activities in common and also many that were unique to the state or local area. All were involved in health education, environmental health, and personal health services, but their orientation toward one or another varied. One emphasized education and environmental inspections, while another concentrated on personal services. Nonetheless, personal health services, particularly for indigent citizens, tended to be a dominant concern in nearly all of the states and local areas.

A fuller description of assurance activities in two states illustrates two methods for fulfilling the assurance function. In one state, the state health agency had a wide variety of programs, including many in health planning and regulation. The state provided much technical assistance and some financing to largely independent local health agencies. In the local area visited in this state, the health agency focused its efforts on sanitation, inspection, and licensing programs. The local agency also offered home health services and provided immunizations and some health screening. Personal health services in the local area were provided by a separate family health center, run by the city health and social services agency; a public hospital; and several special not-for-profit clinics, such as a family planning clinic and a methadone maintenance clinic. There were also numerous private physicians in the area, as well as several not-for-profit and for-profit hospitals.

In the second state, the state health agency also provided a range of programs, but concentrated on personal health services. The local health agencies in this state were run by the state health agency. A variety of personal health services were offered by local health agencies, including maternal and child health, screening, immunizations, ambulatory care, and home health. Activities in education and environmental health took place, but were less emphasized. Some private home health services and not-for-profit community health centers existed, but the public health agency provided personal health care for a majority of the low-income citizens.

Specific illustrations of health programs in which the states and local agencies were involved are numerous. These programs involved both health agency efforts and cooperative ventures between health agencies and other participants in the health system. In education, three states were working fairly intensely on AIDS education programs for both the public and the at-risk groups. In one of these states, the legislature had dedicated funds for AIDS education, and 14 local health agencies had applied to receive funds. In two of the states, citizen groups were involved in AIDS education efforts. In the third, a nonprofit drug rehabilitation clinic was also involved. Two local areas were beginning education programs in schools on family planning and adolescent health. In one of these areas, the local health agency was seeking foundation funding to establish a school-based clinic with comprehensive services for adolescents, which it hoped would be a model for other schools. One state agency was providing education in the school system on smoking and had also set up a hotline for environmental information. One local agency was providing dental health education. Another had a consortium involving representatives from different public agencies and citizens for education on alcoholism.

In environmental services, one state and two local agencies were involved in improving water supply quality. One state agency was devoting considerable resources to asbestos removal in public schools, and two states had special initiatives to clean up hazardous waste sites.

In personal health services, two states were attempting to increase immunization efforts. One was concerned with controlling a rise in measles cases. The other was encouraging rural mothers to bring their children in for immunization at an earlier age rather than waiting until entrance into school. Many local agencies were providing prenatal care and home health services to elderly house-bound citizens.

Each of the six states had systems for providing health services to indigent residents. One provided a majority of the indigent care in its local health departments and in private and charity hospitals. Another provided indigent care mostly in community clinics, as well as in the county health departments, and had a special fund for care provided in private hospitals. A third financed all care in private and university hospitals through its reimbursement system. In this state, hospitals received a percentage above the base rate equal to the percentage of indigent citizens served. A fourth state agency provided finances to county health departments and community clinics to provide indigent care. This state provided 70 percent of the anticipated costs of providing this care directly to the counties, which were by law responsible for medically indigent adults, and directly funded about 100 local primary care clinics, which served primarily minority populations. A fifth state had a catastrophic care fund delegated by the state legislators and by each county. Citizens could apply to their county executive for reimbursement of expenses under $20,000, if they could prove need. For expenses above $20,000, state funds became available. The last state was developing a set of basic services to be provided by public or private clinics and financed by the state. The commission designing the program was hoping to provide a package of basic preventive health care services for a cost to the state of $50 per person per month. Several other strategies for state support of indigent care were discussed during open meetings of the committee.

Despite all of these various programs, there were many examples of health problems for which services were not being offered by health agencies or by other participants. One state was facing a crisis in obstetrics care. In this state, 14 counties had no obstetric services for poor women. Many physicians were refusing to accept Medicaid patients because they felt that Medicaid rates for this service were insufficient in light of the costs of their malpractice insurance. In one local area, no mental health and substance abuse services were available, notwithstanding a high rate of alcoholism among the populace. Only one private nonprofit clinic offered mental health care in a multicounty area. In another state, health officials mentioned that they had concerns about smoking, but that nothing was being done about this problem. In another, many children were not receiving dental care.

Several issues concerning the assurance and delivery of health services were mentioned. In regulation, several participants named areas in which standards were insufficient. Many were trying to increase state regulatory activities for specific programs. In one state, the state agency had recently adopted regulations for certifying water systems operators, in order to enforce more strictly water supply regulations. Another state was hoping to develop regulations on the use of medical devices, in order to limit radiation imposed by these instruments. Another had recently revised its reimbursement regulations for subsidizing care for the medically indigent. In many cases, the need for further standards, regulations, and new policies was mentioned.

Some states also described difficulties with setting standards and regulations in new areas and the risk of meeting with public resistance if the agency is perceived as exceeding its authority. One legislative representative said, "You have to prove there's a real danger before limiting liberty." A citizen of another state said, "We want government out of as much as possible." A physician at an open meeting commented that too many regulations infringe on private providers. Yet the committee also frequently heard such comments as "Government ought to be involved in all areas people can't do for themselves, health included."

In delivery of personal health services, the most frequently mentioned problem was unmet need. Every state and local area visited had minority or indigent populations that local health and government officials and the citizens felt were being underserved. Participants in open meetings described problems with unmet need in additional states. A physician at one of the open meetings pointed out that health problems tend to be more extensive and more severe in indigent populations. Citizens lacking health care include migrants, illegal immigrants, homeless people, Native Americans, the elderly, people in remote rural areas, and people in inner city ghettos. The need for better and more health services was voiced repeatedly. A Native American representative in one of the states visited said, "It's frustrating—the health care in Indian Health Service facilities is not anywhere near what's available in the private sector." A health official in another state declared, "We must be clear about the judgment that health care doesn't depend on race, income, or class." Just as frequently, the need for more health education in an entire range of issues was voiced. A health official in a state with a relatively large number of AIDS victims remarked that the agency's entire budget could be spent on AIDS education. Many health officials and providers also mentioned problems with geographic access. The question, said one local health officer in a rural area, is "How much are you willing to pay to have health care within 50 miles?"

The extent of unmet need in many areas caused agencies to be concerned about their responsibility to meet all needs, particularly those of indigent populations. In several of the local areas, other resources for personal services were abundant—in the form of nonprofit clinics, public hospitals, and private practitioners—and the health agency relied on these sources to carry out personal health activities. But in some of the local areas, the health department was one of the few providers of health services, and the agency was having difficulty meeting all needs. Some local agencies mentioned that they have difficulty maintaining preventive, assessment, and environmental services and still provide a large amount of personal services. Other agencies seemed comfortable with both these roles. In a state that provided a majority of the personal health services to its low-income residents, a local health officer said, "We've never questioned providing direct care. Scope may be a problem, but the function is not." Another health official in this state said, "Government has to be responsible for personal health care as well as preventive measures and the environment." But a private provider in a different, but equally economically deprived, state said, "People can't expect the government to provide erection to resurrection coverage." Open meeting participants mentioned that many state governments are unwilling to provide the large amount of funding necessary for providing health care to all indigent people as well as support public health departments.

Agencies also mentioned the difficulty of maintaining vigilance on old problems while addressing new issues. In one state, environmental health officials felt that their effort was unduly focused on dangers of radiation from a possible nuclear reactor accident, although the public was suffering more radiation damage from medical devices. A local agency had difficulty calling state attention to an increase in measles cases and the need for greater efforts in measles immunization, because most state officials assumed that measles epidemics are no longer a problem. Many state and local health officials at open meetings described the need for public health agencies to become more involved in health promotion and the difficulty of doing so while maintaining other programs.

Intergovernmental and Interorganizational Relationships

It is evident in the examples of health agency leadership, assessment, policy-making, and assurance of educational, environmental, and personal health services observed during the site visits that the ability of health agencies to carry out their responsibilities relies in part on their relationships with other participants in the public health system. Many of the activities described above were not and could not be carried out by a local health agency alone. In many cases, the other agencies, private providers, and private associations in the area worked with the public health agency.

Relationships in carrying out public health functions are fourfold: between different health agencies at various levels of government, between health agencies and other public agencies, between health agencies and the private sector, and between various private organizations. As in all other aspects of the public health system, the states showed a range of possibilities in all four types of relationships. Relationships ranged from cooperative to competitive to indifferent. In two states, relationships between the state and local agencies were minimal. The state health officer in one of these despairingly declared, "The key word here is home rule." The other said, "It's almost heresy to say that the state should involve itself more with locals." In another state, the state and local agencies were a single system. In one state, other public agencies with duties relating to health were well organized and coordinated with the state health agency. In another, the agencies did not communicate. In two local areas, many cooperative arrangements existed between private clinics and the health department. In another, private and public clinics maintained a friendly but competitive relationship, and in one local area they virtually ignored one another.

The patterns described above were not even consistent to a state or local area. In some places, relationships between public agencies were minimal, but relationships between public and private providers were strong. Or relationships between organizations would be strong on a particular health issue, but not on other issues. In two of the states, although relationships between the state health agency and local agencies were minimal, considerable networking between state-level agencies took place in one state, and networking between the local agencies and private providers took place in both. In one of these states, environmental agencies collaborated on issues with the state health department, but the mental health agency did not. And the local area had extensive networks for maternal and child health and AIDS, but not for mental health and health care for the homeless.

Numerous examples of successful coordination between public agencies and between public and private agencies were described to the committee. Several local health agencies mentioned that they were receiving assistance from the Centers for Disease Control or special funds from another federal agency. In one state, a board of environmentally related agencies, including health, had been formed to investigate the nuclear waste issue. In one local area, the health agencies of nine counties had joined together and joined with the community clinics in the area to form a consortium for primary health care. The organizer of this consortium was the local health officer for two of the counties. In another local area, the health department had set up a system that included health department clinics and private hospitals for delivering prenatal and obstetrics care to indigent women. In one state, private professional associations and the state legislature and citizen groups had banded together to promote a smoking cessation campaign.

But many interviewees also described situations in which they felt greater coordination would be desirable. In the two states in which the Indian Health Service had facilities, almost no contact was taking place between the federal service and the state agencies. In one of these states, the Indian Health Service, the state health agency, and the state mental health agency were arguing about responsibility for adult and aging services. In another state, numerous environmental agencies existed, all dealing with different environmental issues, and none of them dealing with the health agency. In another local area, most health issues were handled without contact between the health department, the public hospital, and various nonprofit clinics in the area.

Problems associated with communication in the public health system were described. Some agencies felt that relationships between health agencies at different levels of government were more formal than functional. Some health officials even described their relationships as dictatorial. A representative anecdote concerns the state health officer who instituted new regulations defining local health departments without consulting local health departments.

Problems were also mentioned with interagency communication. Several agencies were accused of "turf-guarding." Officials bemoaned the lack of definition among responsibilities, particularly between environmental and public health programs. In one area, the local health officer felt that none of the numerous state environmental agencies took responsibility for local environmental issues, so these problems had been left to the local health department. In one state, the state health agency felt hampered in its efforts to enforce rules on individual water supply, because responsibilities were split with the state environmental agency. Officials also described overlap problems with personal health programs. In one state, the Medicaid agency and the state health department were described as collecting the same information from providers without sharing data. In the states with significant Native American populations, Indian Health Service programs were run completely independently from those of the state. This practice caused difficulties for Native Americans living outside of reservations, and for people who are only partially Native American, who are sometimes denied service by both state and federal programs.

Some problems were also described in health agency communication with the private sector. Many agencies said that cooperation between the public and private sector was imperative. Said a state health agency director, "We have to maintain good relationships with the private doctors; if they won't work with us, we're dead in the water." But some meeting participants said that if the health department relies too heavily on private providers, it can lose control of programs. Others described competition between public and private providers. Said a state official, "We have a statewide system of home health care—we get a lot of competition from private providers." In this state, the state agency considered competition helpful, but the director of one private home health agency did not. A private physician in one area of the state said, "If the health department routinely refers patients to [another area], they keep on going, and we lose patients." In this same state, the committee heard that a local health agency was not accepting referrals from the local community health center. Participants in the open meetings pointed out that many physicians are unwilling to become involved with the health department because fees for services are so low or funding for programs is cut without warning.

Resources

The six states visited illustrated patterns of financing and difficulties with constrained resources indicated by national trends.

The six states varied in their basic economic situations; in the amount of money their health agencies received from federal, state, and local sources and how these finances were allocated; in the manner in which finances were shared between state and local agencies; in the amount spent on different types of programs; and in their staffing of state and local agencies.

Two of the states visited were among the wealthier in the nation. One was recovering from a recession in the early 1980s, in which large numbers of residents had lost their jobs. Another was beginning to feel severe effects from the current national farm crisis. And two were among the most chronically poor in the nation. The local areas visited followed much the same patterns as their states, although two of the local areas in the wealthier states were substantially less economically well-off than the state average. And one local area was generally better off than the majority of areas in the state.

State per capita health expenditures ranged from $72 to $172 among the six states in 1984. (U.S. Department of Commerce, 1986) Also in 1984, total state and local health agency expenditures ranged from $736 million in the largest, most populated state to $14 million in the least populated state. These figures were $517 million and $13 million for the same states in 1980. (Association of State and Territorial Health Officials, National Public Health Program Reporting System, 1981; Public Health Foundation, 1986)

In 1984, total state and local health agency funding derived from federal contracts and grants ranged from 10 to 60 percent in the six states. Funds from the states ranged from 0 to 60 percent. Local funds accounted for 0 to 60 percent. (Public Health Foundation, 1986; see Figure 4.1) The percentage of federal funds allocated for general administration "core" support in the states ranged from 0 to 2 percent.

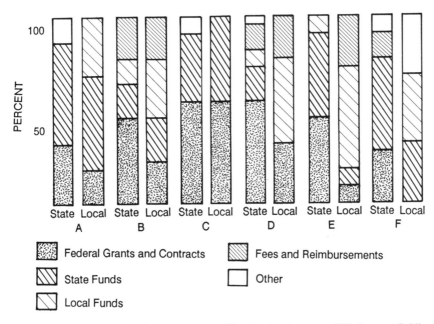

FIGURE 4.1   State and local agency sources of funding for six states, 1984. SOURCE: Public Health Foundation, 1986.

Program expenditures of state and local agencies for different health programs varied throughout the states (see Figure 4.2). For example, agencies spent as much as 95 percent to as little as 45 percent of their budgets on personal health services. Within this, funding for specific services varied. For example, in two of the states that were similar in population size and economy, one of the state agencies spent $1.6 million on health statistics activities, while the other spent $500,000. In communicable disease control, one spent nearly $8 million and the other spent $860,000. In maternal and child health services, one spent $52 million and the other spent $20 million. (Public Health Foundation, 1986)

Finances from health agencies were not the only source of funding for health programs. Individuals in states and localities frequently mentioned finances from other sources. Sometimes special programs had been arranged with additional grants from federal sources. Sometimes funding had been received from private foundations. For example, one local area had a community-based program for AIDS victims financed by The Robert Wood Johnson Foundation. In one state, the Appalachian Regional Commission had assisted with many programs. In all of the states, health care providers as well as agencies mentioned Medicaid, Medicare, and Social Security as

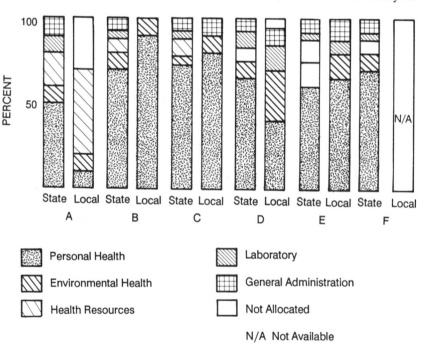

FIGURE 4.2 Areas of expenditure of state and local health agencies in six states, 1984. SOURCE: Public Health Foundation, 1986.

sources of finances. And public health spending also took place in environmental, mental health, social service, and agricultural state agencies.

In staffing, the state agencies ranged in number from 312 full-time employees to more than 4,000. In four of the states, the number of agency staff was remaining fairly constant. One state was planning a large increase in staff in one particular program. Another had lost a small number of staff.

The number and type of professional staff varied between agencies. One state agency had only one physician in the agency, the health officer, who filled an advisory role to the director. Another health agency had a physician with a master's degree in public health heading nearly every program. One of the states had physicians from the U.S. Public Health Service working in the agency. One local area had a physician from the National Health Service Corps. Most of the state agencies had a large number of nurses on staff; in one of the agencies, nurses made up nearly a quarter of the staff. Each of the states had only a few health educators. Planners, data analysts, and statisticians generally made up less than 10 percent of the staff in all of the six state agencies. In three of the states, environmental personnel made up about 10 to 20 percent of the staff. (Association of State and Territorial Health Officials Foundation, 1985)

Staff of the local agencies ranged from a few dozen to more than 600. The smallest had no physicians on staff; the largest had several. All of the agencies had several nurses on staff; a few had health educators; most had sanitarians. All had at least one administrative staff person. Only the larger agencies had separate staff for vital statistics activities. The number of staff was fairly constant in most localities.

In most of the areas, the populace relied on private health care professionals to provide services as well as on health agency staff. The number of public health professionals and health care professionals in the states and localities working outside of the public health agencies varied; physicians per 1,000 population ranged from 107 to 230 in the six states. (U.S. Department of Commerce, 1986) Two of the states had public health schools within the state. Each state had at least one medical school. And each had at least one nursing school. In the local areas, the numbers of private physicians ranged from three or four to a county in the most rural sites to hundreds in the large cities. Nurses ranged from only a few to several hundred. And hospitals and clinics ranged from dozens to only one or two to a county.

Several states were engaged in special activities in resources development. One had a governor's conference on wellness. Another had raised special federal funds for high-risk maternity care, and the agency in this state was also encouraging physicians to accept jobs in underserved areas and training pediatricians and nurses in high-risk maternal care. One state agency had obtained funding from a private organization to start up an insurance program for small employers. And another was seeking funding for research on the numbers of and health needs of illegal immigrants to the state. One state had a special program for training and hiring physicians specializing in preventive medicine.

The most frequent problem mentioned concerning resources in site visits was the lack of funds to support ongoing and new health programs. This problem was reiterated throughout open meetings. Although state and local agency people in the sites did not complain a great deal about past budget cuts, a general lack of finances was frequently mentioned. Many felt that departments could not adequately fulfill all of their responsibilities because of lack of funding. A state health official said, "You know you'll get blamed if things go wrong, but no one will give you the money to help you get ready." And a county supervisor described their dilemma, "We rob Peter to pay Paul just to put out the fires." Several health officials mentioned programs or activities that were in danger of being cut because of lack of funding. A local health officer told the committee, "The county hospital pays for ambulance service, but it's losing money—we can operate the service through next year, but after that. . . ." A clinic director in the same local area, a rural county with a large migrant population, said, "Refugee money will be ending this year—I don't know how we'll continue to provide services." Public health officials also described limiting programs because of financial ability. A state health official said, "First you define a problem, and then you decide if you can afford it." A local health official in an area with high infant mortality rates told the committee, "The high-risk pregnancy program is limited in number due to funds." And a public health agency clinic administrator confided, "We constantly prescribe less expensive medications or put off tests." Many health officials and providers mentioned concern about increasing indigent care and uncompensated care in their states. Some officials feared further cutbacks. A state health officer declared, "If revenue sharing goes down, 22 local health departments will have to close." One of these local health departments said it had no alternative but to shut down if federal funds were lost. Several other departments mentioned the need to seek funding for programs from other sources. One state health officer said, "In a poor state we have to look at wherever we can find the funds—we can't sit back and decide this is impossible, now bring us the money for it." Some also mentioned a lack of staff. In one local agency, the local health officer felt that his abilities had been severely limited by loss of a key colleague. Participants in open meetings also mentioned problems with staff shortages.

A few site visit residents mentioned concerns about training public health personnel. They mentioned that training should include political and communication skills, as well as scientific and technical skills. One state health officer said, "Public health training is narrow and disciplinary, not outcome oriented. We say we're scientists, not politicians." A public health professor said, "We need to teach people to say 'ten leading cripplers and killers,' not morbidity and mortality." The difficulties of providing education that both trains frontline workers and educates leaders was extensively discussed at one of the committee's meetings. The need to interest medical school students in public health and preventive medicine was mentioned at another open meeting. The committee also noticed that the training and background of officials in state and local health departments visited varied tremendously. In some agencies, most officials had training in medicine, public health, nursing, health education, or a related field. But in some agencies, few had public health-related training. Many had spent long careers in public health, but some had no public health experience prior to employment in the agency.

CONCLUSION

The above description of the public health system is meant to highlight its diversity and its dynamism. The system is a problem-processing activity, involving many participants in different settings and in different disciplines, who deal with similar and with individual problems. The variety throughout the system is a consequence of the different values and participants present in each area and of how these participants determine problems, make decisions about needs, and organize and allocate resources to meet needs.

Autonomy and the right to make independent relevant decisions about needs in local areas is a fundamental American approach to government. But there are also values, equally fundamental, that support the need for government to provide or make available core public health functions and activities to all citizens. These values and issues were discussed in Chapter 2 of this report. Observation of the current public health system, as described in Chapter 4, shows that some states and some local areas are more able to fulfill these functions than others. Some far exceed the minimum, but some don't meet it. The following chapter evaluates the current system as described and considers problems and opportunities for bringing the current system, as a whole, closer to the ideals expressed in Chapter 2.

REFERENCES

American Medical Association, Department of State Legislation, Division of Legislative Activities. 1984. *State Health Departments*. American Medical Association, Chicago, Ill.
Association of State and Territorial Health Officials Foundation. 1985. *Staffs of State Health Agencies*. ASTHO Foundation, Washington, D.C.
Association of State and Territorial Health Officials, National Public Health Program Reporting System. 1981. *Public Health Agencies, 1980: A Report on Their Expenditures and Activities*. ASTHO, Washington, D.C.

Bureau of Data Management and Strategy, Health Care Financing Administration. 1985. *HCFA Statistics*. U.S. Department of Health and Human Services, Washington, D.C.

Council of State Governments. 1985. *The Book of the States, 1984–5*. Council of State Governments, Lexington, Ky.

Council of State Governments. 1987. *The Book of the States, 1986–7*. Council of State Governments, Lexington, Ky.

Executive Office of the President, Office of Management and Budget. 1987. *Budget of the United States Government, Fiscal Year 1988*. Government Printing Office, Washington, D.C.

Grad, Frank P. 1981. *Public Health Law Manual: A Handbook on the Legal Aspects of Public Health Administration and Enforcement*. American Public Health Association, Washington, D.C.

Hanlon, G., and J. Pickett. 1984. *Public Health Administration and Practice*. Times Mirror/ Mosby.

Miller, C. Arden, and Mary K. Moos. 1981. *Local Health Departments: Fifteen Case Studies*. American Public Health Association, Washington, D.C.

Miller, C. Arden, E. F. Brooks, G. H. DeFriese, B. Gilbert, S. C. Jain, and F. Kavaler. 1977. "A Survey of Local Public Health Departments and Their Directors." *American Journal of Public Health* 67(10):931–39.

Omenn, G. S. 1982. "What's Behind Those Block Grants in Health." *New England Journal of Medicine* 306(17):1057–60.

Public Health Foundation. 1986. *Public Health Agencies, 1984*, vols. 1, 2, and 4. Public Health Foundation, Washington, D.C.

Public Health Foundation. 1987. *Public Health Agencies, 1987*. Public Health Foundation, Washington, D.C.

U.S. Department of Commerce. 1986. *National Data Book and Guide to Sources: Statistical Abstract of the United States*, 106th ed. Government Printing Office, Washington, D.C.

5

Public Health as a
Problem-Solving Activity:
Barriers to Effective Action

Carrying out the public health mission described in Chapter 2 requires systematic identification of health problems and the development of means to solve those problems. This volume has described the history of the development of this problem-solving capability and its current status in the United States. With that description as a backdrop and drawing on a review of the literature, site visits, statements at the four open meetings, review of other case studies (Miller and Moos, 1981; Institute of Medicine, National Academy of Sciences, 1982b), and the recent evaluation of progress by the U.S. Public Health Service—*The 1990 Health Objectives for the Nation* (Office of Disease Prevention and Health Promotion, Public Health Service, U.S. Department of Health and Human Services, 1986), the committee has identified some appreciable barriers to effective problem solving in public health. These barriers include:

- lack of consensus on the content of the public health mission;
- inadequate capacity to carry out the essential public health functions of assessment, policy development, and assurance of services;
- disjointed decision-making without necessary data and knowledge;
- inequities in the distribution of services and the benefits of public health;
- limits on effective leadership, including poor interaction among the technical and political aspects of decisions, rapid turnover of leaders, and inadequate relationships with the medical profession;
- organizational fragmentation or submersion;
- problems in relationships among the several levels of government;

- inadequate development of necessary knowledge across the full array of public health needs;
- poor public image of public health, inhibiting necessary support; and
- special problems that limit unduly the financial resources available to public health.

Unless these barriers are overcome, the committee believes that it will be impossible to develop and sustain the capacity to meet current and future challenges to public health while maintaining the progress already achieved. Deaths and disabilities that could be prevented with current knowledge and technologies will occur. The health problems cited in Chapter 1, and many others, will continue to take an unnecessary toll, and the nation will not be prepared to meet future threats to health.

Public health faces the simultaneous challenges of responsiveness and continuity. Sustained successes frequently lead to apathy, and the visibility and excitement surrounding new problems promote ad hoc decisions that fragment programs and divert resources from established and successful programs.

This chapter concentrates on identification of barriers most needing attention, thereby setting the agenda for the recommendations to follow. Emphasis on barriers rather than accomplishments may seem to cast public health in an unduly negative light. Public health has a record of accomplishment that should be a source of pride. Yet problems that can erode current and future capacities of public health should be identified and faced if public health is to continue its record of accomplishment.

THE LACK OF CONSENSUS ON MISSION AND CONTENT OF PUBLIC HEALTH

Progress on public health problems in a democratic society requires agreement about the mission and content of public health sufficient to serve as the basis for public action. There is no clear agreement among public decision-makers, public health workers, private sector health organizations and personnel, and opinion leaders about the translation of a broad view of mission into specific activities. As described in Chapter 4, the governmental activities that can be described "public health" vary greatly among jurisdictions. This diversity reflects a wide variety of views about the appropriate scope of public health activities among the many publics that must support public health in the political process and through supportive activities in the private sector. Thus, it is difficult to build effective constituencies that extend beyond a particular issue to the support of broad purposes and the necessary continuing infrastructure of public health.

In our interviews we found many examples of constituencies formed around specific issues (for example, toxic waste disposal, AIDS, Alzheimer's disease, promotion of healthful life-styles, improvement of infant mortality rates). A democratic society favors organization of action around specific issues, an American tendency identified by De Toqueville in the middle nineteenth century. (De Toqueville, 1899) Although such a specific focus often generates political support for action, it can also contribute to disjointed and fragmented decisions, to lack of concern with longer-term issues, and to lack of support for a more comprehensive vision of the public health mission. Without a coherent and widely shared view of public health, it is difficult to translate specific interests into sustained support for a broader public health capacity.

In addition to the diversity of activities among state and local jurisdictions described in Chapter 4, the committee identified several particular issues that divide public health.

PUBLIC HEALTH RESPONSIBILITY FOR INDIGENT CARE

Some public health workers are concerned when their agencies serve as providers of last resort for medical care of the indigent, or administer Medicaid or other financing programs. Those concerned see these functions as detracting from essential public health activities such as disease surveillance and control through prevention. One county health officer told us that "when you put together preventive and curative, the latter gets the money, because no one has the guts to say I'm going to emphasize prevention. Sickness care takes precedence."

Others see the public health role in the care of the indigent as essential—at least until other means are devised by society to take care of these needs. In many of our site visits, we were told of overwhelming unmet needs for medical care of the indigent. As noted in Chapter 4, almost three-quarters of state and local health agency expenditures are for personal health services. Many public health agencies have a long-standing focus on the provision of maternal and child health services to the indigent, emphasizing those services that have substantial long-term benefit through disease prevention and health promotion. (Miller and Moos, 1981; Public Health Foundation, 1986) This maternal and child health focus has been especially strong in a number of public health agencies in the South.

The tension caused by attempting to provide personal medical care services without at the same time depriving other public health functions of an appropriate share of scarce funds is aggravated by overall changes in the financing of medical care, which force more of the burden of care of the indigent back on to public agencies. (Desonia and King, 1985) Because the dollar flow for medical services is large, and because reimbursement through federally matched sources of funding, such as Medicaid, is available, care of the indigent looms large in the state budget-setting process as compared with other public health functions. Identification of public health with care of the indigent in the minds of decision makers and of the general public sometimes clouds the perception of the importance of public health to the entire population. For example, in one state the committee visited, the state health department pays for more than one-third of births each year. This, plus a strong family planning program, has contributed to an impressive reduction in the state's infant mortality rate in recent years. Yet this record does not win the public support that it should: the well-to-do either don't know about the department's services to the poor or see them as unrelated to their own needs. The state's legislature voted more funds for Medicaid, then cut the health department budget. By contrast, in a Canadian city visited during the study, universal entitlement to medical care lifts the burden of indigent care from the public health agency, leaving that agency free to focus its resources on other priorities in public health, such as effects of industrial pollutants on cancer incidence, improving the health outcomes of high-risk infants, smoking cessation, monitoring health status, and organizing the community to combat particular health problems.

Relationship of Public Health to Environmental Health

Many of the early accomplishments in the prevention of infectious disease were accomplished through public health management of water supply and sewage disposal. Even though a certain degree of tension existed from the earliest days of public health between environmental health activities relying heavily on sanitary engineering techniques and surveillance by sanitarians and the work of public health physicians and nurses providing preventive services to individuals, environmental health activities were integral parts of public health services until the 1960s and 1970s. Then major changes occurred in environmental health policy, planning, and organization at both state and federal levels of government. (Rabe, 1986) This movement combined a concern about such issues as protecting natural resources and energy conservation with the traditional environmental health activities designed to reduce the risk of disease and dysfunction. Many advocates of stronger public actions to prevent contamination of the environment saw existing public health agencies as too slow in responding to the need for new actions.

One effect of this increased public attention and the perception of unresponsiveness from public health agencies was a splitting off of many environmental health concerns from public health activities. The split was symbolized at the federal level by the creation of an independent new agency—the Environmental Protection Agency—to administer programs concerned with air and water, solid waste, pesticides, noise, and ionizing radiation. Most of these programs had once been a part of the Public Health Service. A similar organizational change took place in states. (Hanlon and Pickett, 1984; Rabe, 1986) The implications of these changes are considered later in this chapter, but a notable effect was to separate public health from the broad-based constituency interested in environmental protection. Those environmental protection functions still within the operational purview of public health, such as food protection and enforcement of standards for drinking water quality, were not as well supported and as well publicized as were programs for the control of pesticide use and for the reduction of human exposure to air pollution or ionizing radiation. Responsibility for identification, education, and modification of important environmental factors that increase the risk of illness and premature death was separated from other interrelated public health functions. As a result, many observers believe, the health implications of environmental hazards have not received the depth of analysis or the level of support they deserve. In some cases, uninformed analysis of environmental health risks may have exacerbated fears of those risks unnecessarily.

RELATIONSHIP OF PUBLIC HEALTH TO MENTAL HEALTH

During most of its long history, the public function in mental health primarily was on care of the chronically ill mental patient, as illustrated by the large hospitals for the mentally ill. This activity in personal health services contrasted with the usual public health focus on prevention of disease and protection of the health of the public. Differing perspectives and operating modes were often reflected in organizational separation of mental health from public health at the state level. At the federal level, mental health responsibilities remained within the Public Health Service, although mental health groups have advocated the maintenance of a separate identity for mental health programs both at the state and federal levels in order to assure sufficient attention to these important health problems.

The trend in mental health services in the United States since World War II has been away from large custodial institutions and toward community-based services, stimulated by the National Mental Health Act of 1946 and by the federal Community Mental Health Centers legislation in the 1960s. This community approach and the mental hygiene movement, which had its origins in this country, were based on the belief that mental health problems were related to the community context, not only to the individual. (Turner, 1977) Thus, epidemiological concepts began to be applied to the identification of mental health problems in the population, and an interest in prevention of mental illness, promotion of mental health, and the early diagnosis of mental problems began to parallel more closely the traditional concerns of public health. Many health problems, such as those stemming from substance abuse, accidents, family violence, and teenage pregnancy, were recognized as having behavioral underpinnings.

Despite this expansion of the range of mental health services to include many public health issues, the relationship between public health and mental health remains underdeveloped. Organizational, historical, professional, and interest group barriers to more productive interaction persist even though mental health and public health have moved closer together conceptually.

The need for a community-based strategy for prevention in mental health, drawing on fundamental public health concepts, was recognized by the Joint Commission on Mental Illness and Health in 1961 and the President's Commission on Mental Health in 1978. (Joint Commission on Mental Illness and Health, 1961; President's Commission on Mental Health, 1978) Referring to the progress made by public health in preventing disease and promoting health, the President's Commission stated that "The mental health field has yet to use available knowledge in a comparable effort." (President's Commission on Mental Health, 1978) The strategy they recommended would be based on identification of high-risk groups in the population, identification of factors contributing to those risks, and development of cost-effective means of intervention to reduce risks, consistent with this society's community and individual values. This strategy is consistent with the public health vision outlined by this committee in Chapter 2.

THE PUBLIC HEALTH ROLE IN ENCOURAGING HEALTHFUL BEHAVIORS THROUGH EDUCATION AND THROUGH MODIFICATIONS IN THE SOCIAL ENVIRONMENT

Many of the modern opportunities for health improvement lie in achieving life-style and behavior changes. The evidence linking health problems to behavior is extensive. Well-known examples include links between lung cancer and smoking; AIDS and sexual behavior; motor vehicle trauma, teenage driving habits, and alcohol consumption; and family violence linked to family and job-related stress.

Educational efforts to tell persons about health risks or healthful behavior have been used to effect desired changes. Many of these efforts have been carried out by the private sector, often using the public media or private educational programs (e.g., advertising campaigns by voluntary health organizations). The role of state or local public health agencies has often been relatively minor. In the site visits, we often found that efforts to achieve healthful behavior did not seem to occupy a prominent place on the public health agenda.

In addition to intervention to change individual behavior, other strategies seek to control factors in the "social environment." However, health programs to educate youth about the dangers of tobacco and alcohol, for example, are rarely matched by efforts to reduce consumption of these substances by increasing taxes or controlling advertising. Although public health professionals have traditionally recognized influences of the *physical* environment on health status, they have been less adept at recognizing health-related influences in the business, economic, and social environment and in fashioning and advocating strategies to control these factors.

Yet, in spite of the need for further definitive research, considerable evidence now demonstrates that the social environment can be a major cause of illness. (Institute of Medicine, National Academy of Sciences, 1982a; Berkman and Breslow, 1983) Job and family stress; promotion of hazardous products; encouragement of risk-taking behavior and violence through TV programs, movies, and other popular media; and peer pressure for substance abuse, premature sexual behavior (with associated health risks of sexually transmitted disease and teenage pregnancies), and school failure all are potential or actual etiologic factors in health problems, both physical and mental. Public health programs, to be effective, should move beyond programs targeted on the immediate problem, such as teen pregnancy, to health promotion and prevention by dealing with underlying factors in the social environment.

To deal with these factors, the scope of public health will need to encompass relationships with other social programs in education, social services, housing, and income maintenance.

IMPEDIMENTS TO THE ESSENTIAL WORK OF PUBLIC HEALTH

In its investigations, the committee found a number of problems impeding the ability of those charged with public health responsibilities to carry out the essential functions of assessment, policy development and leadership, and assurance of access to the benefits of public health.

ASSESSMENT AND SURVEILLANCE

A foundation stone for public health activities is an assessment and surveillance capacity that identifies problems, provides data to assist in decisions about appropriate actions, and monitors progress. Epidemiology has long been considered the essential science of public health, and a strong assessment and surveillance system based on epidemiologic principles is a fundamental part of a technically competent public health activity.

Federal agencies, such as the Centers for Disease Control, the National Center for Health Statistics, and the National Institutes of Health, have provided national leadership, data, and technical assistance, all of which assist states and localities in carrying out their assessment responsibilities. However, many states and localities lack a fully developed capability for this essential function. While the collection of vital statistics has long been a state responsibility, other critical data are available only in the form of national sample surveys that cannot be directly desegregated to state and local areas without significantly compromising their accuracy. Table A.4 in Appendix A tells, for example, that half of the states collect morbidity data and even fewer conduct health interview surveys. On the other hand, the collection of data about communicable disease, health screening for some specific problems, and laboratory analysis are functions conducted by essentially all of the states.

The level of support provided for the function of assessment and surveillance reflects these difficulties and the competition for limited resources with other more publicly visible public health priorities. For example, in one state the committee visited, vital statistics had not been published at all during the 2 years preceding our visit. In another, a county health officer reported having to wait more than 2 years for aggregated data from the state after sending in local birth and death statistics.

Achieving and sustaining a comprehensive and integrated assessment and surveillance capacity is made more difficult by the fragmentation of the assessment function in many states where environmental health and mental health data are gathered by separate agencies. Meanwhile, the lack of direct federal encouragement and assistance to state efforts has limited the availability of good health data at the state and local levels.

POLICY DEVELOPMENT

Policy development is the means by which problem identification, technical knowledge of possible solutions, and societal values join to set a course of action. The site visits and other information available to the committee raise many issues about the soundness of current policy development in public health.

Much good work has been done at the national level in generating health data, in analyzing and applying those data to public health problems, and in the development of planning tools like *The 1990 Objectives for the Nation* and *Model Standards*. (U.S. Department of Health and Human Services, Public Health Service, 1980; American Public Health Association et al., 1985) However, in the site visits and other inquiries, we found that policy development in public health at all levels of government is often ad hoc, responding to the issue of the moment rather than benefiting from a careful assessment of existing knowledge, establishment of priorities based on data, and allocation of resources according to an objective assessment of the possibilities for greatest impact.

The resulting pattern of policy decisions, which has been described as a "successive limited comparison" or as disjointed and "incremental" (Lindblom, 1959), is well established in the American public decision process, reflecting, perhaps, our national penchant for immediate problem solving, belief in the desirability of limited government, and widespread distrust of government "social planning." Policy development can follow the interests of charismatic decision-makers (sharp examples were offered in the site visits of the influence of particular legislators or county commissioners on a particular issue) without adequate consideration of options, unintended side effects, long-term results, or effective allocation of resources based on impact on health status. Although *The 1990 Objectives for the Nation* and *Model Standards* serve as very good frameworks for objective setting and systematic policy formulation, we saw little evidence of knowledge about or use of these planning tools in our discussions with state and local decision-makers. In fact, as the director of the Medicaid agency in one state observed, policy is too often decided on the basis of single cases. During the time we visited that state, the plight of an uninsured woman in need of a heart–lung transplant was monopolizing public dialogue, while severe stress-related problems among the state's farmers and their families—alcoholism, family violence, accidents—received little notice even among public health professionals.

Another problem is the fragmentation of policy development because of governmental structure. That structure is discussed in greater detail later in this chapter, but it deserves mention here because of its impact on policy formulation. Some of the fragmentation and diffusion of public health policy development is inherent in the U.S. system of government with its separation of powers between executive, legislative, and judicial branches and its federal system of national and state governments with further delegation by the states to local jurisdictions. In addition, health-related responsibilities are frequently divided among several agencies at the federal, state, and local levels (see Appendix A). The result is multiple decision-makers on a given issue, diffusion of responsibility and accountability, delays in decisions, and unresolved conflicts. We should also note, however, that a diversity of decision-makers may create opportunities for initiatives and innovations, for closer tailoring of policies to local circumstances, and for constituency groups to find an action point for a particular issue.

In a society that historically has preferred to minimize the role of the public sector, the committee finds that there is often a lack of a clear rationale for the public provision of services in the policy development process. It is not sufficient for the policy process to identify a need and a technical means to address the need. The policy determination also should include consideration of the appropriate public and private roles in which the public purpose is made clear, regardless of whether public or private means are chosen for conduct of the activity. The scope of public health often includes objectives that can be and are accomplished through stimulation of private actions rather than through direct public provision of services. In our interviews, several persons observed that public agencies often seem more comfortable with direct conduct of activities than with more indirect modes of action, such as stimulation of private activity to accomplish the public objective.

The relationship between the public and private sectors for the accomplishment of public health objectives becomes particularly apparent when regulation is the mode of public health activity chosen through the policy development process. Here again, a clear identification of the public purpose in the policy development process is necessary, along with the technical underpinning that can be provided by a solid assessment function. (Committee on the Institutional Means for Assessment of Risks to Public Health, Commission on Life Sciences, National Research Council, 1983) Sound analysis of health risk in the development of regulatory policies (e.g., water and air pollution controls, food safety, licensing of health providers) can lead to more rationality and credibility in the final regulatory decisions. It also can better concentrate public effort on activities that will lead to the greatest reduction of health problems for the effort and funds invested. The recommendations of the recent Institute of Medicine report on the regulation of nursing homes is an example of the link between a public assessment function and desired private actors. (Institute of Medicine, National Academy of Sciences, 1986) The importance of health risk analysis has also been recognized in the recent Federal Appeals Court decision holding that, in assessing the impact of proposed regulations, the Environmental Protection Agency must consider potential health risks rather than potential costs as the overriding factor. (*National Resources Defense Council* v. *Environmental Protection Agency,* 1987)

One by-product of a systematic policy development process is the identification of gaps or uncertainties in the knowledge base that should guide decisions.

Some problems with the policy development process can be accentuated through the domination of the process by very narrow special interests. For example: the board of health in one state consists entirely of representatives of the state medical society. Other special interests may dominate through the activities of key legislators, county commissioners, or appointments to public health leadership positions on the basis of narrow political interests. The final determinations in public health should always be political in the sense of being responsive to broad public values, but the committee is concerned that particular decisions—especially those with important technical content—may not have passed through a technically competent policy development process.

Another limitation on the development process is a constraint on the ability to respond to new challenges. This constraint may result from limited funding for public health activities or from the structure of budgetary decisions (e.g., 2-year budget cycles, limits on shifts among budget line items, Propositions 13 and 4 in California, Gramm–Rudman–Hollings at the federal level). Such structural boundaries on the decision process can hamper response to new challenges (e.g., AIDS, toxic waste disposal) by forcing substitution of the new activity for old functions. Added to the typical inertia of any organization and budget, these negative pressures put a special strain on the policy development process. In theory a good policy development process should be just as important for deciding on program reductions as it is for determining desirable program expansions. In practice, a ratchet effect is often observed in which it is much easier to consider program expansions on top of existing activities than it is to consider realignment of programs according to program priorities.

ASSURANCE OF ACCESS TO THE BENEFITS OF PUBLIC HEALTH

Assurance of the availability of the benefits of public health to all citizens reflects a primary reason for the existence of *public* health activities. The committee identified many problems that impede the achievement of that assurance.

As described in Chapter 4 and Appendix A, the committee observed very wide variation of the content and intensity of public health activities across the country. Because benefit from well-conceived public health activities is clearly established, this variation means that there is considerable inequity in access to these benefits from jurisdiction to jurisdiction, as well as by social and income status. Decentralization of decisions and funds from the federal level accentuates this inequity, as does decentralization within states to local jurisdictions. For example, in one county visited, all the obstetricians–gynecologists in the county had unilaterally declared that they would no longer provide prenatal care to Medicaid or other poor patients. This was partly a protest against low reimbursement rates and partly an effort to pressure the state to do something about skyrocketing malpractice costs. Whatever the reason, the effect on poor women was devastating: they had literally nowhere to go for prenatal care since the health department did not provide such services. Women were presenting in labor at the local emergency room, having not seen a physician during their entire pregnancy.

Concern about equity implies that wide access to specified benefits is desirable. Within a nation of diverse needs, resources, and political structures, some diversity in the patterns and intensity of public health services is expected and appropriate. However, the committee was concerned about the degree of this diversity. A diverse response to local needs and circumstances needs to be balanced, in the committee's view, with sufficient attention to equity of access to the benefits of public health programs. The degree of diversity of public health services in the country indicates that states and communities lack agreement on those services to which access should be assured.

Although *Model Standards* can be important tools for establishing a basic level of assurance, they leave wide leeway for states and localities to define their own version of extent of assurance of such public health benefits. (American Public Health Association et al., 1985) The objectives established by the Public Health Service, with considerable participation of other elements of the society, imply the desirability of universal access to the benefits of public health. (U.S. Department of Health and Human Services, Public Health Service, 1980) As indicated in Chapter 1, and as shown in the considerable progress toward achieving the objectives for 1990, even more equitable distribution of public health benefits is a realistic goal for many problems. (Office of Disease Prevention and Health Promotion, Public Health Service, U.S. Department of Health and Human Services, 1986) The success in controlling some communicable diseases is so dramatic as to constitute a benefit that is universally available. The benefits of other public health interventions are more inequitably distributed. An effective assessment system that provides surveillance at the state and local level is necessary to identify inequities, especially for health problems such as injuries or chronic diseases for which the availability of services is more uneven and the role of public health less clearly established. Yet these problems loom large as causes of premature death and disability. Achieving desirable public health objectives such as smoking cessation, limiting the transmission of AIDS, prevention of low birthweight, and control of human exposure to toxic substances raises complex political and value issues in which the protection and improvement of the health of the public conflicts with other social values, such as individual freedoms or economic growth. The conflicts may erode support for effective public health actions, leaving gaps in access to benefits.

A special problem in assuring access to the benefits of public health activity is the diversity of funding sources for public health activities. Financial support for public health services varies greatly from state to state even after including federal block grant and project funds provided to the states (see Appendix A). In some states the amount of state and local funding is so minimal that basic services are heavily dependent on a flow of dollars from reimbursement by private and federal sources. Implicit in a concern about achieving assurance under present conditions of wide variation is a willingness of higher levels of government—federal and state—to reallocate tax revenues to areas of greatest need.

LEADERSHIP FOR PUBLIC HEALTH

In its inquiries the committee found a number of problems that limit effective leadership for public health. The committee's vision for the future of public health requires leaders whose skills encompass a wide range of necessary characteristics, including technical competence in the substance of public health issues; managerial abilities; communication skills; knowledge of and skills in the public decision process, including its political dimensions; and the ability to marshall constituencies for effective action. The committee recognizes that this is a demanding and multifaceted characterization of the desirable leadership skills, and, as in most complex organizations, the efforts to identify individuals with potential for leadership and to develop and nurture these capacities will be an ongoing challenge that often falls short of the ideal. However, the committee believes that more attention needs to be given to overcoming the specific problems that inhibit effective leadership. The following are specific problems that we identified.

THE INTERACTION OF TECHNICAL EXPERTISE AND POLITICAL ACCOUNTABILITY

In exploring the making of public health decisions in particular states and localities, we observed that technical expertise bearing on some public health problems may not be appropriately considered by the political policy-makers, leading to decisions that are technically inadequate. For example, policymakers may not appreciate the problems raised by false positives in a testing program that is screening a low-risk population. The controversy over mandatory testing for AIDS sometimes reflects this lack of understanding. On the other hand, we observed that the technical experts may not understand or appreciate the appropriate and fundamental role for the political process in public policy-making, especially as it expresses society's values as criteria for selecting among options that have been defined with appropriate technical competence.

CONTINUITY OF LEADERSHIP

In many public health jurisdictions, rapid turnover of leadership has been a problem. For example, the median tenure of state health officers in 1987 was about 2 years. (Gilbert et al., 1982) This rapid turnover probably reflects political–technical conflict, inadequate pay, the effects of reorganization, frustrations with the structure of decision-making, and low professional prestige. A rapid turnover of political appointees in federal, state, and local government is an established pattern in the American political system, reflecting the high value Americans place on making their government responsive to the democratic process. However, for an activity like public health, which is based on technical knowledge, rapid turnover of leadership in key positions can erode desirable technical competence. We have observed a trend in some jurisdictions to make key public health positions more subject to appointment on primarily political grounds than on the basis of professional expertise and standing, using "responsiveness" to new policy directions as a rationale. In one state the committee visited, political appointees occupy the top three levels of the health department hierarchy. When the governor changes, much of the leadership of the agency is wiped out. In this instance, career employees seem to be regarded as liabilities instead of assets, that is, the governor is widely reputed to see them as holdovers from the previous administration.

Another factor in the discontinuity of leadership has been the decline in the role played by the U.S. Public Health Service Commissioned Corps in providing experts on assignment to state and local public health agencies. For decades, the Commissioned Corps provided a personnel system with retirement benefits that allowed assignment of corps officers to state and local positions, constituting a national cadre of trained public health personnel. Although still used for this purpose, the corps membership has declined and has been less available for state and local assignment. (U.S. Public Health Service, Health Resources and Services Administration, 1987)

NATIONAL LEADERSHIP FOR PUBLIC HEALTH

The provision of appropriate national leadership for public health is closely related to the problems of governmental structure in our federal system as discussed earlier. The components of necessary national leadership include (1) identifying and speaking out on specific health problems, (2) allocating of funds to accomplish national public health objectives, (3) building constituencies to support implementation of appropriate actions, and (4) supporting development of the knowledge and data base by public health. The federal government has been active in all of these components over the years. The role of the Centers for Disease Control in strengthening the public health capacity of the nation is apparent and profound. The establishment of the Office of Disease Prevention and Health Promotion in the Public Health Service provided additional focus on public health issues. Publication of *Healthy People* (U.S. Department of Health, Education, and Welfare, 1979) in 1979 and the subsequent issuance of *The 1990 Objectives for the Nation* (U.S. Department of Health and Human Services, Public

Health Service, 1980) and of *Model Standards* (American Public Health Association et al., 1985) represented a visible national leadership role in the establishment of public health objectives, working with state and local agencies and state and national nongovernmental health groups. The Environmental Protection Agency has played a major role in reducing environmental pollution. The National Institutes of Health led the campaign against hypertension. The National Institute of Mental Health led in the development of community mental health resources. The leadership role of the Surgeon General and the Public Health Service in reduction of smoking has been essential. Many other examples could be cited.

There have been complaints from state and local agencies since the 1960s that the federal government sometimes bypassed them in carrying out some federal health priorities. Examples include health planning, community health centers, regional medical programs, and professional standards review organizations. However, the current federal policy stance, going back over several administrations, has been to turn over more public health decision-making to the states. This has been accompanied, however, by a reduction in the flow of federal funds earmarked for public health activities, measured on an equivalent current services basis. For example, when the public health, mental health, and maternal and child health block grants were approved by Congress during the sweeping changes in 1981, decision-making was transferred to the states, but the federal funds included in the block grants were cut by 25 percent. (Omenn, 1982) Some national policy-makers argued for elimination of federal support for these functions. At the same time, federal revenue sharing was being eliminated, thus further reducing available federal funds that could be used for public health purposes. While some restoration of federal revenues was made by Congress in 1983, a net reduction from prior levels is still in place.

The AIDS epidemic has demonstrated the need for federal leadership in public health. Only the federal government can focus the attention and resources that such a health problem demands. In our site visits, many state and local officials welcomed national leadership on such issues, but at the same time complained about the fragmenting effect of some federal policies and programs and the lack of resources to carry out federal requirements.

POOR RELATIONSHIPS WITH THE MEDICAL PROFESSION

A particular problem for public health leadership is the lack of supportive relationships with the medical care profession. There are numerous examples of practicing physicians being supportive of public health activities, but confrontation and suspicion too often characterize the relationship from both sides. The director of one state medical association perceived the state health department (led by a nonphysician) as failing to seek medical advice and as distrustful of private physicians. He cited the department's effort to get a mandatory data reporting system through the legislature without consulting the association. On the other hand, health department personnel—including the director—told us that it was impossible for the department to do its job without the support of private physicians. As one official put it, "Without them, we're dead in the water." In contrast, we heard of one local health officer who, confronted with the problem of access to prenatal care, convened a meeting of local obstetricians to ask them each to agree to take one or two patients for whatever they would pay. The doctors all agreed, and the problem was resolved.

We found medical care leaders who were simply unaware of the activities carried out by public health; yet those same leaders are often crucial in the achievement of political support for public health activities and in the conduct of substantive public health activities in which the cooperation of the private medical community is highly desirable (e.g., the reporting of communicable diseases, the provision of prenatal care, the education of the public on healthful personal habits, and many other examples). Improving these relationships is an important challenge for public health leadership.

COMMUNITY ORGANIZATION FOR PUBLIC HEALTH ACTION

In a free and diverse society, effective public health action for many problems requires organizing the interest groups, not just assessing a problem and determining a line of action based on top-down authority. There are many positive examples of public health officials taking leadership in organizing community support for actions toward public health objectives, but this dimension of leadership is not as firmly fixed in public health activities as may be desirable. This capability requires appropriate leadership skills and techniques, as well as an attitude that the community itself is a source of public health actions. These skills include the ability to communicate important agency values to public health workers and to enlist their commitment to those values, the ability to sense and deal with important changes in the community that are the context for public health programs, the ability to communicate with diverse audiences and to understand their perspectives and needs, and the ability to find common pathways for action. Appropriate training in these leadership skills needs to be a part of the educational preparation of public health leaders.

STRUCTURE AND ORGANIZATION OF PUBLIC HEALTH

In the United States, public sector functions must be performed in the midst of a deliberately complex set of organizational and jurisdictional relationships. Policymakers and decision-makers are multiple, and organizational arrangements reflect both constitutionally determined layers of government and the multiple interests in a democratic society competing for attention and resources. Coherence and consistency of function are very difficult to attain and sustain under these circumstances. The following are specific problems we have identified.

ORGANIZATIONAL SEPARATION OF ENVIRONMENTAL HEALTH PROGRAMS, MENTAL HEALTH PROGRAMS, AND INDIGENT CARE PROGRAMS

In a previous section, we discussed the problems that are created for a perceived coherence of public health activities when environmental health, mental health, and indigent care programs are administered by separate agencies. These separations also raise administrative, structural, and policy questions. In the case of environmental health, the committee was presented during its site visits with tangible indications of barriers to action caused by fragmentation of responsibility. In one county, officials were concerned about several toxic spills on highways, one of which had occurred near the county's open reservoir. They had written more than a year prior to our visit to the state attorney general, who had jurisdiction in such cases, and as yet they had no answer. In another state, a rancher showed us the notebook of correspondence he had amassed over several years of attempts—as yet unsuccessful—to dispose legally of two barrels of toxic waste on his property.

Concern was also expressed that organizational fragmentation lessens desirable health-related technical input into the policy- and decision-making process—especially for environmental health activities and for the Medicaid program when it is administered by a social services agency. For mental health programs, the organizational separation may reflect a continued emphasis within mental health on the provision of services for the mentally ill rather than a "public health" orientation, including epidemiological surveillance and prevention.

Wherever organizational separation takes place, regardless of the validity of the reasons for that separation, separate program development is encouraged and desirable program coordination is impeded. Data systems are fragmented, impeding broad assessment and surveillance that make possible comparisons of program impacts on the health of the public and policy formulation based on comparable problem analysis and risk assessment. In the committee's judgment, this separation contributes to the sense of disarray in public health that inhibits coherent governmental effort to improve and protect the health of the public. Such separation also divides constituencies that might otherwise help develop a broader vision of the public health mission.

CREATION OF HEALTH AND HUMAN SERVICES SUPERAGENCIES

As described in Appendix A, almost half of the states have created umbrella health and human services "super" agencies. This combination of health and welfare accentuates the image in the minds of some policymakers that public health is predominately a welfare program. As a result, the relevance of public health to the broader society may be diminished. The emphasis of such health and welfare agencies on the coordination of services to particular individual clients, although a worthy objective, may give less attention to the broad population-based functions of public health that benefit the entire public.

Another problem with these umbrella health and human services agencies that was described to us is the appointment to managerial positions in these agencies of administrative generalists, with little or no health background or expertise. Desirable inputs from technically competent persons may therefore be subordinated in the policy and administrative process. Generalist managers may also be less attuned to a broad vision of public health, such as that set forth by this committee in Chapter 2.

It should be noted that at the federal level the Public Health Service has been part of such a "super" health and human services agency since before World War II (until 1977 also including education).

From the perspective of advancing a public health mission, the committee notes that both in the fragmentation model described above and the superagency model, the role of public health leadership founded on a technically competent assessment function is lessened. Case studies have been made of these organizational changes (Lynn, 1980), but we note that there is no solid evidence of the impact of alternative organizational patterns on health status. Nevertheless, on the assumption that organizational structure can enhance or inhibit some aspects of program effectiveness, the committee believes the structural issues deserve attention.

We also believe that whatever the organizational structure, coordination with other human services programs will be necessary. For example, many issues of policy and program coordination will continue to exist at the interface between social programs and public health programs, especially for multiproblem families or vulnerable individuals, such as the disabled or the frail elderly. Likewise, such programs as housing, land-use planning, criminal justice, and education have important health implications. Public health will always have to reach across organizational boundaries for health-related inputs on policies and programs, just as other agencies will have to seek appropriate inputs from health agencies on their policies and programs. We question whether the "super" agency health and welfare model has been a useful solution to those coordination needs.

LACK OF A CLEAR DELINEATION OF RESPONSIBILITIES BETWEEN LEVELS OF GOVERNMENT

The federal structure established in our Constitution deliberately introduces a degree of ambiguity and tension concerning the roles of the various levels of government. This ambiguity can clearly be seen in public health where we observe a "patchwork quilt" of relationships.

Questions about the appropriate division of responsibilities will probably persist as long as we have a federal structure of government. However, the committee is concerned that the lack of a clearer delineation of those roles impedes desirable cooperation and optimal use of the unique capacities peculiar to each level. Some patterns of relationship, such as the relationship of the Centers for Disease Control with states and localities in the control of communicable disease, seem to be relatively clear and productive. For other functions the relationships are less well established and are often sources of considerable tension. In the 1960s, the federal government deliberately bypassed official health agencies at the state and local levels in establishing certain federal health programs, such as neighborhood health centers and regional medical programs, to assure that federal objectives were met. Some environmental health problems raise complex questions of interstate or even international relationships in which a purely state or local focus of authority is insufficient for the problem. For example, in one of our site visits a county commissioner pointed out that pollution of beaches in his jurisdiction was caused by sewage effluent from a foreign country that borders on his district.

The relationship between the state and localities is extremely varied and is a product of particular provisions of state constitutions, political history, and inherent tensions between large urban areas and rural areas within a state. In most states, the statutes describing the authority of and relationships between state and local health agencies lack clarity and consistency. Often these statutes consist of successive overlays on prior law, rather than comprehensive codifications. Previous grants of authority to village, town, city, county, and state health officers and boards may have been made at different times using inconsistent language, resulting in a confusing patchwork of law which often mirrors an equally ambiguous set of relationships in practice. These ambiguities are often reflected in poor communication and in understandings between state and local officials.

This complex of problems deserves explicit attention if the future of public health is to be assisted by appropriate cooperation rather than impeded by dispute and confrontation.

DEFICITS IN THE CAPACITY TO CONDUCT PROGRAMS

In carrying out its functions, public health must possess the fundamental capacity for effective actions. These capacities include the technical knowledge base and its application, well-trained and competent personnel, the generation and maintenance of adequate constituencies and political support, managerial competence sufficient for these complex public sector tasks, and adequate fiscal support for the agreed-upon public health mission. The committee has identified problems with each of these capacities.

KNOWLEDGE AND ITS APPLICATION

Effective public health actions must be based on accurate knowledge of health problem causation, distribution, and the effectiveness of interventions. Actions often must be taken on the basis of incomplete knowledge, but these knowledge gaps can impede effectiveness of programs and ultimately public support for actions. For many public health problems the knowledge base, including knowledge about the effectiveness of specific interventions, is inadequate. Arguments in the policy formulation and regulatory decision processes often question knowledge that does exist, e.g., human health risks of toxic chemicals or effects of smoking on nonsmokers. Filling these knowledge gaps requires substantial resources, yet the need for additional knowledge is often perceived by decision-makers only when the decision needs to be made. Public health may then be accused of lacking competent expertise relevant to the immediate needs of decision makers.

Another problem with filling these knowledge gaps is the extraordinary breadth of substantive areas that are relevant to public health actions. Some knowledge arenas such as epidemiology are obvious, but public health is also a primary beneficiary of advances in biomedical knowledge that lead to definitive interventions, such as the development of new screening tests and vaccines. The research response to the AIDS problem illustrates this relevance. The same can be said for toxicological research that improves the ability of public health to perform informed risk assessments. The incredible ferment in research that is adding to our basic understanding of biological processes is, therefore, highly relevant to public health, as is reflected by the conduct of such research in a number of schools of public health.

Other knowledge bases are not quite so obvious but, nevertheless, important. For example, the recent report *Confronting AIDS* noted the importance of behavioral research, including fuller knowledge about sexual behavior, as an essential component of a successful public health strategy to limit the spread of this dread disease. (Committee on a National Strategy for AIDS, Institute of Medicine, National Academy of Sciences, 1986) Also relevant is evaluative research drawing on the social sciences in determining the effectiveness of public health interventions, both retrospectively and prospectively.

Because public health is an applied activity—usually carried out under firm fiscal constraints—it is often very difficult to nurture and sustain the necessary research activities in support of the public health effort. In our six site visits, we found only one state that made a substantial investment in research. It may be logical to aggregate much of the research effort to the federal level as has traditionally been done; however, this may leave undeveloped the function of applied research as a link between a generation of new basic knowledge and its application in the field. Private foundations have played a valuable role in the demonstration and education of new public health approaches. Just as developments in clinical practice have been enhanced by the conduct of clinical research, so it is essential that public health be enriched by appropriate basic and applied research in the full range of sciences relevant to public health.

THE NEED FOR WELL-TRAINED PUBLIC HEALTH PERSONNEL

Many sections of this report have mentioned the need for well-trained public health professionals who can bring to bear on public health problems the appropriate technical expertise, management and political skills, and a firm grounding in the commitment to the public good and social justice that gives public health its coherence as a professional calling. The committee has identified a number of problems in meeting this need. Most public health workers, including some public health leaders, have not had formal educational preparation focused primarily on public health. (Institute of Medicine, Conference, March 1987) Those with adequate technical preparation may lack the training in management, political skills, and community diagnosis and organization that is appropriate for leadership roles in a complex, multifaceted social service activity. Public health leadership also requires an appreciation of the processes and values of government in the United States. The continuing evolution of public health constantly raises new challenges to public health personnel, requiring updating of knowledge and skills.

Many educational paths can lead to careers in public health, but the most direct is to obtain a degree from a school of public health. Schools of public health were established in major private universities early in the century. They now number 25—7 in private universities and 18 in public. During the early decades of their existence, they concentrated on training people with degrees in the health and related professions (physicians, nurses, engineers, dentists, and others) to become public health professionals. In recent years, however, as the mandate of public health has broadened and as public health problems and their solutions have become more complex, the schools have responded to this evolution by recruiting individuals from the behavioral sciences, from mathematics, from the biological sciences, and from other relevant fields and disciplines, as well as health professionals. (Institute of Medicine, Conference, March 1987)

Modern schools of public health serve important dual roles: that of a public health research institute and that of a public health educational facility. These roles reflect the great successes of public health in developing new knowledge and applying that knowledge in a social and political context to the benefit of the population. The complexity of modern issues in public health requires that the field continue to develop new technologies delivered in new ways. These technologies require both fundamental and applied research before they can be implemented as public health programs in an agency setting. Schools of public health have traditionally operated to serve this basic and applied research function, linking knowledge generation with practical problem solving. Meeting the challenges to public health described in this report will require a strengthening of this linkage. The schools can build on their previous efforts to work cooperatively with agencies in evaluating public health programs and in assisting in their initial implementation.

Many schools of public health are located in research universities and therefore have specific responsibilities to the academic objectives of their institutions as well as to their fields of professional practice. This situation is by no means limited to public health, but characterizes graduate professional education in medicine, dentistry, engineering, law, and other fields. Each of these areas must accept the dual responsibility to develop knowledge and techniques of use to the profession and to produce well-trained professional practitioners.

Many observers feel that some schools of public health have in recent years become somewhat isolated from the field of public health practice. The result of this changing emphasis may be that some schools no longer place a sufficiently high value on the training of professionals for work in health agencies. The variation in public health practice noted earlier in this report and the limitations on employment opportunities in health agencies for well-trained professionals, restricting opportunities for graduates, have inhibited desirable responses by the educational institutions to the needs of practice. This situation is exacerbated by the fact that most public health workers have not had appropriate formal professional public health training. However, we lack sufficient knowledge about the public health workforce and its needs and opportunities.

Recognizing the importance of these and other issues relating to the education and training of public health personnel, the committee sponsored an invitational conference in Houston in March 1987 in cooperation with the University of Texas School of Public Health. The conference brought together public health educators, practitioners, and other concerned individuals to consider the future of education and training for public health. It helped identify issues, clarify consensus and areas of disagreement, and provide a broader input into the committee's deliberations. The proceedings of that conference will be published separately from this report.

DISTRIBUTION OF TECHNICAL EXPERTISE

Technical expertise in public health is not evenly distributed among jurisdictions. Some of the larger states have considerable internal expertise. Others lack such expertise. The consultation role of the Centers for Disease Control and the larger state public health agencies help fill this need, but important gaps remain. For example, in one of the states we visited, an assignee from the Centers for Disease Control was carrying out an important epidemiological study. When his short-term assignment was completed, however, the expertise necessary for essential assessment activities was no longer present on the staff. Public hearing participants reported that cutbacks in federal staffs, especially at the regional office level, have reduced the federal consultative capacity. This problem is further exacerbated by the lack of trained experts in such fields as epidemiology. Previous studies have shown persistent deficits in their availability. (Institute of Medicine, Conference, March 1987) In some jurisdictions, low salaries and unrewarding professional environments would inhibit the attraction of such expertise even if a sufficient aggregate supply existed.

BUILDING CONSTITUENCIES FOR PUBLIC HEALTH

Our inquiries indicate that public health seems to suffer from a poor image or lack of attention even when its success in the solving of specific problems is highly publicized and commended. We were told by state and local elected officials that the general population often cannot identify the benefits they have received through public health activities. Public health, in this regard, suffers from its successes. Such achievements as a safe water supply, the disappearance of many childhood infectious diseases, reduction of the incidence of stroke, fewer childhood poisonings, reductions in lead poisoning, and control of food-borne infections are taken for granted until a problem occurs. Also, the identification of public health programs with means-tested welfare programs adds to the perception that public health concerns are not an integral part of the entire community.

Some of the public may have additional negative views of public health based on perceived interference with private freedoms and a moralistic tone of public health pronouncements. For example, smokers may resent efforts of public health authorities to limit smoking in public places. Other important interest groups, such as the tobacco industry, may oppose public health actions and question the competence of public health agencies because those actions may interfere with the economic interests of the group.

Although the broader medical community can and does identify with such public health issues as smoking, injury control, infectious disease control, and dietary change related to cardiovascular disease and cancer, many physicians look down on public health, as an organized activity, believing it to be second rate or meddlesome. The one-on-one orientation of most medical training, the limited exposure to such population-based concepts as epidemiology, and the lack of experience during the training process with interdisciplinary collaboration contribute to this lack of a natural alliance between the physicians and public health.

Finally, public health has both an enforcement (negative) and a facilitative (positive) aspect. This sends mixed signals about the image of public health to various population and interest groups.

We identify image as a problem not because we are concerned about the sensitivities of public health workers, but because we believe that these problems interfere with the capacity of public health agencies to mobilize the support of important constituencies, including the general public, for the public health mission. The image problem may also limit recruitment of talented persons into the field of public health practice. In a free society, public activities ultimately rest on public understanding and support, not on the technical judgment of experts. Expertise is made effective only when it is combined with sufficient public support, a connection acted upon effectively by the early leaders of public health.

MANAGERIAL CAPACITY

We have identified many aspects of the needed managerial capacity in the previous discussions, specifically under the label of leadership. Here, we reemphasize the complexity of the managerial tasks faced by the public health manager. We cannot think of a managerial responsibility that involves a wider range of skills, including not only the usual management and leadership skills for running a complex and interdisciplinary organization, but also the communication and constituency building skills of a public executive, and finally, but not least, access to up-to-date technical information, sometimes in emergency circumstances. The high visibility and intense public interest that arises when a public health emergency occurs adds to the stress of these positions. Finally, the nature of public health decisions often places the manager at the center of a conflict among competing societal values and political forces.

The early progress of public health in this country was advanced by the fortuitous presence of individuals who combined these many managerial characteristics. The present challenge is how to assure the ready availability of managers with these capabilities. This is unlikely to occur without special attention and a plan for the development and support of a cadre of talented persons with appropriate educational preparation and experience. Leadership development would be aided by adequate salary levels, particularly in the case of state and local health officers (the current low salaries for many of these positions are documented in Chapter 4 and Appendix A). Modernizing benefit programs so that personnel could accept "promotions" involving a change of political jurisdiction without losing accumulated pension funds would also help with the career development of a management cadre.

THE LACK OF FISCAL SUPPORT

The wide array of challenges facing public health and the strongly ingrained American belief in limited government make it unlikely that adequate financial support for public health activities will ever be available. In the competition with other important public functions, it is probably naive to think that the "right" distribution of available public funds exists. However, we would note these special problems for public health as compared with other public functions:

- an explicit reduction of federal support for public health activities;
- the special financial problems faced by particular states as a result of declines in their economies;
- the appearance of new challenges to public health such as AIDS or the hazardous by-products of modern economies;
- the advance of our techniques both biological and epidemiological to identify risks to human health;
- the changing demographics of American society (e.g., an aging population);
- an interconnected world that shares health risks with increasing rapidity;
- the need to maintain and replace expensive public infrastructures for health, such as water and sewage systems;
- the rise in the costs of modern health care, which both add to the burden on public provision of health services and compete with funds for other public health functions;
- the need to provide sufficient core support for a public health delivery system; and

● the complex requirements and limited rewards for public health managers.

This list could be expanded, but these problems illustrate the challenge of achieving adequate fiscal support for public health activities.

HOW THE PUBLIC HEALTH SYSTEM WORKS—AIDS AS AN EXAMPLE

What are the problems public agencies are having in fulfilling their unique functions—of assessment, policy development, and assurance? Is the statutory base adequate to cope with a new and compelling issue? The intent of this section is to illustrate some of the problems by focusing on one, acquired immune deficiency syndrome (AIDS), and tracing through the system, largely by means of quotations obtained in our site visits.

STATUTORY BASE

According to Gostin (Gostin, 1986), the statutory base of public health is poorly suited to dealing with AIDS. The powers provided in statute are too restrictive, including outdated concepts of full isolation and quarantine that are inappropriate given the mode of transmission of AIDS. Also there are no clear criteria to guide officials in exercising their powers. Due process procedures are sketchy or absent. This leaves too much room for unfettered administrative discretion about how to apply the law. A modern public health law should remove the rigid distinctions between venereal and communicable disease and should enact strong, uniform confidentiality procedures. Otherwise, public health is left with a stick too big to wield.

Site visit comments bear out this view. For example:

"This state has strange confidentiality laws that make it difficult to target appropriate information to appropriate recipients."

"In the legislature there is inordinate emphasis on the physician's lack of information. They're not confronting the position the doctor faces in informing people and their contacts about the disease—for instance, the wife of an AIDS patient. They tried to make knowing donation of infected blood a crime, but it didn't go anywhere."

"Our law has made AIDS a reportable disease. We have little in the way of confidentiality. The new law makes knowing transmission of AIDS second-degree murder."

ASSESSMENT

Exercise of the assessment function is closely linked to the enabling structure put in place by statute. Public health officials feel keenly the need to monitor the disease and mount effective programs to limit its spread. Pursuing these functions raises many political sensitivities. In addition, the speed with which the problem developed has public health struggling to keep up with changing dimensions and new technologies. This makes long-range or even rather short-range planning a luxury agencies can't afford. Some health agencies are accused of overemphasizing surveillance at the expense of preventive efforts such as education.

"The state has taken a commanding lead. They are secretive about sharing stats. I don't want names, but they'll only give out information on a countywide basis. The hospitals are also tight lipped. The vital statistics give us the deaths."

"We're skeptical about the individuals themselves revealing the information. We need to track sero-positive individuals and maintain confidentiality."

"The gay rights groups are concerned about list collecting; they are resisting public health moves to get people in for counseling. On the other hand, there are scientific concerns about anonymous testing. These are new issues for disease control."

"The Department of Health Services has been so busy getting the new initiative implemented we can't really plan adequately. No one has yet been able to take a broader system view of the AIDS problem. No one is thinking about how to fit the pieces together."

"The research program at the university was good, but the main need now is for technology transfer. The results are not getting into the hands of community physicians fast enough."

"The department is trying to use the STD (sexually transmitted disease) model, emphasizing surveillance and epidemiology. I would argue that prevention should take precedence."

POLICY DEVELOPMENT

AIDS is extraordinarily controversial, and the political heat has been intense. Pressure to do something fast, but not to infringe on the rights of high-risk groups, has health agencies struggling to balance basic knowledge development with the obligation to respond to immediate situations. Among the many groups and individuals, public and private, engaged in fighting AIDS, health agencies have not taken a clear initiative in supplying leadership, and the public is unclear about what level of government it should look to for guidance or what it can appropriately and realistically expect any particular health agency to do. Lack of public understanding about the real nature of the risk makes matters worse; on the other hand, as one person said: "If they knew they had practically no chance of getting it, then they really wouldn't give a damn."

"It was publicity that finally raised the consciousness of the eighth floor [health department leaders]."

"The legislature has been the leader. It convened the hearing and put funding in place. Such leadership should have come from the Department of Health Services, but it hasn't. The department has held no hearings. The state health director knows less than I do about what's happening in the state." (Legislative staff)

"The president and the governor should have taken the lead, but they seem not to want to discuss it. At the federal level, only CDC and NCI have been effective." (Activist)

"AIDS dictates the entire public health program in the state to an inappropriate degree. I spend one-third of my time on it. Don't ask me what we're doing about diabetes or high blood pressure. I simply don't know."

"There's not enough attention being paid. What gets done depends on the public mood. Much better education of the general public is needed so they will accept future expenditures."

"In the end, the lack of responsible public health organization for the nation will prove our greatest handicap. Governments, too, can suffer a wasting disease; the gradual erosion of the coordinated leadership of the Public Health Service has created a void. Surveillance of the nation's health is no longer the clear responsibility of any agency of government, nor is the surveillance of proposals for meeting crises. Isolated islands of excellence [CDC, NIH] do not alone constitute a national strategy to defend and promote the national health." (Keller and Kingsley, *The Milbank Quarterly,* 1986)

ASSURANCE

Public health officials at the state and local level are very much aware of their responsibility to make sure that AIDS is combated effectively. But they are hamstrung by the speed with which the problem has developed and the political heat it has generated, as well as by the difficulty of marshalling enough resources to do what they feel is needed. At present, they lack the technology either to cure AIDS or to control its spread through the definitive and simple means of a vaccine. The fiscal implications of caring for AIDS patients are poorly understood because estimates of the potential number of cases are in dispute. In some places where there are large numbers of AIDS patients, the private sector—especially voluntary groups such as gay rights organizations—have taken the lead in providing treatment and counseling, with the health department struggling to keep track of what is being done. The nature of the problem makes the regulatory apparatus difficult to mobilize.

THE STATE OF PUBLIC HEALTH

This discussion of how the public health system is coping with the AIDS epidemic illustrates many of the problems encountered by these agencies when confronted by such a major new challenge. Other examples would have revealed different sets of problems, such as how to sustain a continuing effort to maintain high rates of childhood immunizations where prior success breeds complacency, liability concerns raise the price and threaten the availability of vaccines, and limited resources are diverted to new challenges. Both types of examples, the new crisis and the continuing effort, support a central theme of this report—the essentiality and proved effectiveness of public health measures for improving and protecting the health of the public and the imposing array of problems that undermine the public health capacity to respond. AIDS illustrates both—a strain on the public health system and remarkable accomplishments by the public health community in a short time. Response to a highly publicized crisis like AIDS cannot serve as the model for a sustained and effective public health effort addressed to the many health problems that, in the aggregate, dwarf the health impact of AIDS. For example, the great increase in lung cancer took place more slowly and therefore lacked the dramatic impact of AIDS on the public consciousness, but it is a larger problem in terms of death and disability, and sustained public health effort can affect the magnitude of the disease burden. The same is true for such major sources of health deficits as injuries, substance abuse, and environmental pollutants.

That public health accomplishes so much is a tribute to the effectiveness of its techniques and the dedication of its workforce. Yet the problems and disarray that we have documented through our inquiries are a source of strong concern to the committee. The next chapter contains our recommendations to help overcome these problems, strengthen the public health capability, correct the disarray, and refocus public health on its important mission.

REFERENCES

American Public Health Association, Association of State and Territorial Health Officials, National Association of County Health Officers, U.S. Conference of Local Health Officials, Department of Health and Human Services, Public Health Service. 1985. *Model Standards: A Guide for Community Preventive Health Services*. American Public Health Association, Washington, D.C.

Berkman, Lisa F., and Lester Breslow. 1983. *Health and Ways of Living: The Alameda County Study.* Oxford University Press: New York.

Committee on the Institutional Means for Assessment of Risks to Public Health, Commission on Life Sciences, National Research Council. 1983. *Risk Assessment in the Federal Government: Managing the Process.* National Academy Press, Washington, D.C.

Committee on a National Strategy for AIDS, Institute of Medicine, National Academy of Sciences. 1986. *Confronting AIDS: Directions for Public Health, Health Care, and Research.* National Academy Press, Washington, D.C.

Desonia, Randolph A., and Kathleen M. King. 1985. *State Programs of Assistance for the Medically Indigent.* Intergovernmental Health Policy Project, Washington, D.C.

De Toqueville, Alexis. 1899. *Democracy in America.* Colonial Press, New York.

Gilbert, Benjamin, Mary K. Moos, and C. Arden Miller. 1982. "State Level Decision-Making for Public Health: The Status of Boards of Health." *Journal of Public Health Policy* (March):51–61.

Gostin, Larry J. 1986. "The Future of Communicable Disease Control: Toward a New Concept in Public Health Law." *The Milbank Quarterly* 64(Supplement 1):79–96.

Hanlon, J., and G. Pickett. 1984. *Public Health Administration and Practice.* Times Mirror/ Mosby.

Institute of Medicine, National Academy of Sciences. 1982a. *Health and Behavior: Frontiers of Research in the Biobehavioral Sciences.* National Academy Press, Washington, D.C.

Institute of Medicine, National Academy of Sciences. 1982b. *Health Services Integration: Lessons for the 1980s, vol. 2: Case Studies.* National Academy Press, Washington, D.C.

Institute of Medicine, National Academy of Sciences. 1986. *Improving the Quality of Care in Nursing Homes.* National Academy Press, Washington, D.C.

Joint Commission on Mental Illness and Health. 1961. *Action for Mental Health.* Basic Books, New York.

Keller, Lewis H., and Lawrence A. Kingsley. 1986. "The Epidemic of AIDS: A Failure of Public Health Policy." *The Milbank Quarterly* 64(Supplement 1):56–78.

Lindblom, Charles E. 1959. "The Science of Muddling Through." *Public Administration Review* 19(Spring):79–88.

Lynn, Lawrence E. 1980. *The State and Human Services.* MIT Press, Boston, Mass.

Miller, C. Arden, and Mary K. Moos. 1981. *Local Health Departments: Fifteen Case Studies.* Public Health Association, Washington, D.C.

National Resources Defense Council v. Environmental Protection Agency. 824 F. 2d 1211 (D.C. Cir., 1987).

Office of Disease Prevention and Health Promotion, Public Health Service, U.S. Department of Health and Human Services. 1986. *The 1990 Health Objectives for the Nation: A Midcourse Review.* U.S. Department of Health and Human Services, Washington, D.C.

Omenn, G. S. 1982. "What's Behind Those Block Grants in Health?" *New England Journal of Medicine* 306(17):1057–60.

President's Commission on Mental Health. 1978. *Report of the President's Commission on Mental Health,* vol. 1. Government Printing Office, Washington, D.C.

Public Health Foundation. 1986. *Public Health Agencies, 1984.* Public Health Foundation, Washington, D.C.

Rabe, Barry G. 1986. *Fragmentation and Integration in State Environmental Management.* The Conservation Foundation, Washington, D.C.

Turner, John B., ed. 1977. *Encyclopedia of Social Work,* 17th ed. National Association of Social Workers, Washington, D.C.

U.S. Department of Health, Education, and Welfare. 1979. *Healthy People: The Surgeon General's Report on Health Promotion and Disease Prevention.* U.S. Department of Health, Education, and Welfare, Public Health Service, Office of the Assistant Secretary for Health, and Surgeon General, Washington, D.C.

U.S. Department of Health and Human Services, Public Health Service. 1980. *Promoting Health/Preventing Disease: The 1990 Objectives for the Nation.* U.S. Department of Health and Human Services, Washington, D.C.

U.S. Public Health Service, Health Resources and Services Administration. 1987. Unpublished data supplied to Institute of Medicine Committee for the Study of the Future of Public Health.

6

Conclusions and Recommendations

Public health in the United States confronts a dilemma. On the one hand, the advances against health problems for which public health was established in this country are largely taken for granted: safe water, substantial protection against formerly epidemic diseases, an infant death rate only one-tenth as high as in 1900. It is difficult to maintain a sense of urgency about these matters, although continuing vigilance is necessary to preserve the gains that have been won. For example, our country's progress in reducing infant mortality has actually slipped: throughout the 1970s, infant mortality declined at an average annual rate of 5 to 6 percent, while from 1981 to 1984, the rate of decline slowed to about 3 percent. (Hughes et al., 1986) Infant mortality has actually increased recently in Detroit, Los Angeles, and elsewhere and remains distressingly high in poor communities. Outbreaks of measles, for which effective immunization is available, continue to occur. The rate of syphilis is rising again. (U.S. Department of Commerce, Bureau of the Census, 1986) But warnings about these events by public health officials are sometimes seen as self-serving.

On the other hand, despite general complacency that the public health job is done, public concern is mounting over new health problems: toxic substances in air, water, and food; cancer and heart disease; drug abuse and teenage pregnancy; AIDS. Excitement about such new health threats often leads to laws, regulations, agencies, and appropriations that bypass the "old" public health. Action is obviously necessary, but the traditional channels are widely regarded as unsuitable.

Thus the dilemma faced by public health is how to take on the new challenges while continuing its work to contain long-existing problems.

138

Public health leaders have not succeeded in making clear that both aspects of public health must be tackled vigorously. All too often, political leaders push short-term "solutions" to various health crises without reference to the knowledge base that exists for sound programs. The general public is confused. The result is a hodgepodge of fractionated interests and programs, organizational turmoil among new agencies, and well-intended but unbalanced appropriations—without coherent direction by well-qualified professionals.

That disarray has stimulated this study and this volume.

The first chapter reflects the committee's sense as the study began that public health was in trouble, that few people knew and even fewer cared, and that those who did care were divided over the nature of the problem and what to do about it. In conducting the study, committee members set aside temporarily their individual views—although not their shared concern—in order to take a fresh look at public health and to develop a common understanding of it. The aim of the study has been to produce a report that examines the total range of public health activity, not simply an assortment of tax-supported programs. The committee sought to identify a set of functions necessary for the protection and advancement of the public's health, to assess difficulties in carrying out these functions, and to recommend specific strategies for improvement.

Judgments about the specific programs that public agencies should undertake or what resources they should command always imply underlying assumptions about the agency's proper mission, scope of concern, and functions. In Chapter 2, the committee sought to make its own assumptions explicit, so that the logic of the ensuing problem analysis, findings, and recommendations would be clear. The committee's own deliberations proceeded along these lines, beginning with clarification of the mission and scope of public health. The committee continued by distinguishing functions and responsibilities that *only* governmental agencies can undertake from those that should be shared with or left to the private sector. Then, weighing its analysis of the existing dilemma of public health, as outlined in Chapters 3, 4, and 5, the committee asked with respect to each issue: Given our definition of public health and what we believe government's responsibilities ought to be, how should this challenge be addressed?

This final chapter, setting forth the committee's recommendations for the future of public health, traces the same path. The committee is making three basic recommendations dealing with:

- the mission of public health,
- the governmental role in fulfilling the mission, and
- the responsibilities unique to each level of government.

The rest of the recommendations are instrumental in implementing the basic recommendations for the future of public health. These instrumental recommendations fall into the following categories: statutory framework; structural and organizational steps; strategies to build the fundamental capacities of public health agencies—technical, political, managerial, programmatic, and fiscal; and education for public health.

THE PUBLIC HEALTH MISSION, GOVERNMENTAL ROLE, AND LEVELS OF RESPONSIBILITY

MISSION

• **The committee defines the mission of public health as fulfilling society's interest in assuring conditions in which people can be healthy.** Public health is distinguished from health care by its focus on communitywide concerns—the public interest—rather than the health interests of particular individuals or groups. Its aim is to generate organized community effort to address public concerns about health by applying scientific and technical knowledge. These concerns include disease prevention and health promotion, encompassing physical, mental, and environmental health. Many distinct and diverse professional disciplines are necessary in this effort, such as nursing, medicine, social work, environmental sciences, dentistry, nutrition, and health education. These professions are unified within public health by dedication to its value system, by the public interest in health, and by its core science, epidemiology—the study of health problems in populations and the factors that affect them.

The mission of public health is more fundamental and more comprehensive than the specific activities of particular agencies. Organized community effort to prevent disease and promote health involves private organizations and individuals, working on their own or in partnership with the public sector. But the governmental public health agency has a unique function: to see to it that vital elements are in place and that the mission is adequately addressed.

THE GOVERNMENTAL ROLE IN PUBLIC HEALTH

The committee believes that governments at all levels have an irreplaceable role to play in assuring conditions in which people can be healthy. This means that federal, state, and local public health agencies have an obligation to assume certain vital functions directly. In the committee's view, these responsibilities cannot properly be delegated to the private sector.

• **The committee finds that the core functions of public health agencies at all levels of government are assessment, policy development, and assurance.**

Assessment

An understanding of the determinants of health and of the nature and extent of community need is a fundamental prerequisite to sound decision-making about health. Accurate information serves the interests both of justice and the efficient use of available resources. Assessment is therefore a core governmental obligation in public health.

• **The committee recommends that every public health agency regularly and systematically collect, assemble, analyze, and make available information on the health of the community, including statistics on health status, community health needs, and epidemiologic and other studies of health problems.** The extent to which information will be generated directly or collected from other sources will vary depending on the size of the agency and of the population served. For example, the federal agency will have a nationwide purview, while smaller agencies may lack sufficient mass of expertise necessary for sophisticated research; thus interagency and intergovernmental cooperation is crucial. Nevertheless, each public health agency at every level of government bears the responsibility for ensuring that the assessment function is fulfilled. This basic function of public health cannot be delegated.

Policy Development

Legitimate public decisions reflect a full examination of the public interest and sound analysis of problems and interventions. Attention to the quality of decision-making about health is necessary so that the interests of all affected parties, especially the general public, are considered. This attention is a basic responsibility of government in public health.

• **The committee recommends that every public health agency exercise its responsibility to serve the public interest in the development of comprehensive public health policies by promoting use of the scientific knowledge base in decision-making about public health and by leading in developing public health policy. Agencies must take a strategic approach, developed on the basis of a positive appreciation for the democratic political process.**

Specific strategies must be developed by each agency depending on its circumstances. Later recommendations exemplify the kinds of steps that agencies may find appropriate. The intent of this recommendation is to encourage agencies to view policy development as central to their roles and to develop strategic approaches to its achievement that anticipate possible problems.

Government should be equipped for this role by the technical knowledge and professional expertise of agency staff. Used judiciously, the knowledge base of public health tempers the excesses of partisan politics and encourages just decisions. Technical knowledge will have the best effect, however, when used in the context of a positive appreciation for the democratic political process, by professionals who are politically as well as technically astute.

Assurance

Government has an inherent responsibility to take positive action to achieve goals that society agrees upon in the interest of individual justice or for the common good.

- **The committee recommends that public health agencies assure their constituents that services necessary to achieve agreed upon goals are provided, either by encouraging action by other entities (private or public sector), by requiring such action through regulation, or by providing services directly.**

The goals agreed upon should be achievable with the resources and techniques available. The goal for assurance of a particular service or benefit, therefore, may represent partial accomplishment of an ultimate goal. However, for a subset of assured services that the society, through government, has decided are so fundamental to the well-being of the population that access to their benefits should be universally available, assurance should become a guarantee.

- **The committee recommends that each public health agency involve key policymakers and the general public in determining a set of high-priority personal and communitywide health services that governments will guarantee to every member of the community. This guarantee should include subsidization or direct provision of high-priority personal health services for those unable to afford them.**

Federal, State, and Local Responsibilities

The committee believes that assessment, policy development, and assurance are obligatory functions at every level of government. But federal, state, and local governments are far from identical. They vary in power, responsibility, scale of activity, and level of resources. Therefore it is appropriate that core governmental functions are differently expressed at each level. Also, the idea that there is strength in diversity is a fundamental American belief, reflected in the great variability from place to place in the distribution of functions among levels of government. Nevertheless, there are important public health tasks particularly suitable to each level.

States

Under the Constitution, states retain all powers not specifically delegated to the federal government. The committee believes that the recent trend toward increasing state government responsibilities is positive in at least one respect: In fulfilling the public health mission, states are close enough to the people to maintain a sense of their needs and preferences, yet large enough to command in most cases the resources necessary to get the important jobs done. During the study, however, the committee observed that many states are not fulfilling this leadership role, and public health activities have lost institutional focus and broad public support.

● **The committee believes that the states are and must be the central force in public health. They bear primary public sector responsibility for health.**

● **The committee recommends that the public health duties of states should include the following:**

—**assessment of health needs within the state based on statewide data collection;**

—**assurance of an adequate statutory base for health activities in the state;**

—**establishment of statewide health objectives, delegating power to localities as appropriate and holding them accountable;**

—**assurance of appropriate organized statewide effort to develop and maintain requisite personal, educational, and environmental health services; provision of access to necessary services; and solution of problems inimical to health;**

—**guarantee of a minimum set of essential health services; and**

—**support of local service capacity, especially when disparities in local ability to raise revenue and/or administer programs require subsidies, technical assistance, or direct action by the state to achieve adequate service levels.**

The Federal Government

Most health issues affect the majority of Americans directly or indirectly. Therefore, the federal government's involvement in national policy development is necessary. It has the obligation to take the initiative in bringing broad public health policy issues to the attention of the nation, to establish a framework within which interstate and national issues can be debated, and to set national health goals and standards of achievement.

● **The committee recommends the following as federal public health obligations:**

—**support of knowledge development and dissemination through data gathering, research, and information exchange;**

—establishment of nationwide health objectives and priorities, and stimulation of debate on interstate and national public health issues;

—provision of technical assistance to help states and localities determine their own objectives and to carry out action on national and regional objectives;

—provision of funds to states to strengthen state capacity for services, especially to achieve an adequate minimum capacity, and to achieve national objectives; and

—assurance of actions and services that are in the public interest of the entire nation such as control of AIDS and similar communicable diseases, interstate environmental actions, and food and drug inspection.

Localities

Localities are clearly creatures of the state in legal terms, yet politically they are a significant force in the development of policy and the allocation of resources. Because of the great diversity in size, powers, and capacities of the many thousands of local governments in the United States, generalizations about their proper functions must be made with caution. Yet everyone actually lives and works in a "locality," and the local level represents the final delivery point for all public health efforts.

The committee understands that there are many thinly populated areas in this country where it may be unrealistic to envision a full-fledged local health department. Nevertheless, the committee fully supports the concept of "a governmental presence [in public health] at the local level" as developed in the *Model Standards*. According to this concept, "every community must be served by a governmental entity charged with . . . responsibility . . . for providing and assuring public health and safety services." (American Public Health Association et al., 1985) In the case of many county and municipal governments this requirement is indeed fulfilled, usually with state financial assistance and sometimes through direct state operation of the local health department (Chapter 4; Appendix A). But where local government is clearly unequipped on its own to meet the operational responsibility for a public health presence, the state must—in cooperation with local officials—take action to establish it.

It is difficult to generalize about what constitutes an adequate operational definition of "a governmental presence at the local level." Clearly, each tiny hamlet in a county whose total population is only a few hundred people cannot maintain an independent free-standing, full-service, local public health unit. Acknowledging this fact, the committee nonetheless finds that:

● **No citizen from any community, no matter how small or remote, should be without identifiable and realistic access to the benefits of public health**

**protection, which is possible only through a local component of the public
health delivery system.**

Definitive statements about the embodiment of the governmental presence at the local level are difficult—for they range from the full-service metropolitan health department, including a municipal hospital and environmental protection capacity with full delegation of responsibility from the state, to the half-day-a-week traveling public health nurse and visiting environmental health worker from the state health department, or even to a telephone or radio communications network.

Although definitive statements about the nature of the governmental presence may be difficult, it is possible to say with some certainty what it is not. When local people cannot find help or even advice to deal with suspected toxic waste; when low-income women have literally nowhere to go for prenatal care; when persons designated as local health officers by the state are ignorant of their official status or are even deceased; when the crumbling, neglected "county health department" behind the courthouse has neither information nor the ability to help citizens gain access to needed primary medical care—all circumstances the committee encountered during its study—one can say positively that government's responsibility for the health of the people is not being met.

● **The committee recommends the following functions for local public
health units:**

  **—assessment, monitoring, and surveillance of local health problems and
needs and of resources for dealing with them;**

  **—policy development and leadership that foster local involvement and a
sense of ownership, that emphasize local needs, and that advocate equitable
distribution of public resources and complementary private activities commensurate with community needs; and**

  **—assurance that high-quality services, including personal health services, needed for the protection of public health in the community are available and accessible to all persons; that the community receives proper consideration in the allocation of federal and state as well as local resources for
public health, and that the community is informed about how to obtain public
health, including personal health, services, or how to comply with public
health requirements.**

FULFILLING THE GOVERNMENT ROLE: RECOMMENDATIONS

In order to carry out the public health mission by fulfilling the governmental roles and responsibilities outlined above, a number of enabling steps must be taken. They fall into three categories. First, certain improvements are needed in the statutory base of public health. Second, the committee recommends several structural and organizational modifications that hold promise for strengthening the framework within which key functions must be carried out. Third, a number of strategies are detailed to improve public health agency capacities for action: technical, political, managerial, programmatic, and fiscal. Finally, the committee addresses needs in education for public health.

STATUTORY BASE

State public health laws are in many cases seriously outdated. Statements of public health agency authority, responsibility, and organizational structure are inadequate to deal with contemporary problems. Procedural safeguards protecting individual rights are frequently weak or absent.

• **The committee recommends that states review their public health statutes and make revisions necessary to accomplish the following two objectives:**

—**clearly delineate the basic authority and responsibility entrusted to public health agencies, boards, and officials at the state and local levels and the relationships between them; and**

—**support a set of modern disease control measures that address contemporary health problems such as AIDS, cancer, and heart disease, and incorporate due process safeguards (notice, hearings, administrative review, right to counsel, standards of evidence).**

STRUCTURAL/ORGANIZATIONAL STEPS

The committee believes that several organizational measures can be taken to improve the fundamental ability of public health agencies to translate their duties into specific, effective action. The committee notes that "reorganizing" is frequently the *first* resort of a beleaguered bureaucracy when in many cases the problem is not truly structural. Reorganizing will not create a policy commitment where none exists; but the right reorganization may enable a commitment to be implemented more effectively. Organizational modifications should form part of a total approach.

Some of the committee's organizational recommendations are specific to a particular level of government; others relate to the nature of appropriate linkages with public health-related concerns such as environmental health, mental health, indigent care, and social services. All are intended as steps to enable governments to perform the vital functions of assessment, policy development, and assurance. They have the additional aim of identifying organizational focal points for public health activity.

States

States are the primary force in public health. It is appropriate for states to delegate service responsibilities to localities when local governments are or can be equipped to carry them out. But states have the ultimate responsibility for the health of their residents. To fulfill this obligation states must take action to establish a clear, organizational focal point for public health responsibility, one that is accountable to the people through the political process, yet one in which expert professional judgment about issues requiring such input is not confounded or obscured by excessively partisan politics or narrow ideology.

• **The committee recommends that each state have a department of health that groups all primarily health-related functions under professional direction—separate from income maintenance. Responsibilities of this department should include disease prevention and health promotion, Medicaid and other indigent health care activities, mental health and substance abuse, environmental responsibilities that clearly require health expertise, and health planning and regulation of health facilities and professions.**

The committee believes that diffusion of primarily health-related functions among different agencies and the organizational linkage of health with a particular set of related activities—income maintenance for low-income populations—has gone too far in many states. The effect of organizational trends toward fractionation or submersion of health concerns during the past 25 years has been the creation of impediments to the use of the assessment function in the development of health-related policies and programs that focus on the most significant threats to the health of the public. While a variety of organizational steps might improve this situation, the committee is persuaded that a forthright organization that puts primarily health-related functions over competent health-oriented leadership is the most direct approach.

The committee observes that in some states it may not be politically feasible to transfer authority for a particular public health-related function to the department of health from another state agency. But the fact that authority is shared with other agencies does not relieve the department of health from its obligation to assure that public health functions are performed. To accomplish this critical objective, in cases of shared authority, the assessment, policy development, and assurance functions can be supported by mechanisms such as an interagency council chaired by the director of the department of health to review health problems and encourage and coordinate multiagency efforts.

• **The committee recommends that each state have a state health council that reports regularly on the health of the state's residents, makes health** policy recommendations to the governor and legislature, promulgates public health regulations, reviews the work of the state health department, and recommends candidates for director of the department.

The committee notes that whereas 25 years ago nearly all states had boards of health, many of which had responsibilities similar to those it envisions for state health councils, today half the states have dissolved their boards. (Gossret and Miller, 1973; Gilbert et al., 1982) There has been little research on the factors underlying this development. Whatever sound reasons there may be, the committee believes that the disbanding of state boards has meant the loss of an important resource for public health policy. The state health councils should not be means for control of health matters by health professionals, as has occasionally been true of state boards of health in the past. Rather, a council should be a positive framework within which community values and professional knowledge can be blended to reach wise policy judgments that will assure the conditions in which people can be healthy. The committee believes that lay citizens should be in the majority of the membership. To give weight to the body, both lay citizens and health profession members should have considerable stature in the state and be widely perceived as wise leaders.

• **The committee recommends that the director of the department of health be a cabinet (or equivalent-level) officer. Ideally, the director should have doctoral-level education as a physician or in another health profession, as well as education in public health itself and extensive public sector administrative experience. Provisions for tenure in office, such as a specific term of appointment, should promote needed continuity of professional leadership.**

It is often argued that all officials at the agency head level should serve at the pleasure of the governor to assure accountability to the governor's program. We believe that the desirable objective of accountability needs to be balanced with appropriate concern for continuity of competent professional leadership for a set of functions in which the governor, the legislature, and the society as a whole will expect knowledge and experience when the health of the public is on the line. The committee therefore has recommended appointment of a specific term as a means of meeting both the objectives of accountability and appropriate continuity. For example, the health department director might be appointed for 4 years, with the possibility of renewal. To assure orderly transition between governors, the term might begin 1 year after the governor takes office. Other variations of this approach might be developed to accomplish this purpose, but the committee believes that its specific recommendation should focus attention on an important issue.

• The committee recommends that each state establish standards for local public health functions, specifying what minimum services must be offered, by what unit of government, and how services are to be financed. States (unless providing local services directly) should hold localities accountable for these services and for addressing statewide health objectives, using the *Model Standards: A Guide for Community Preventive Health Services* as a guide.

Localities

Local government variations will determine the exact balance appropriate between direct state operation of local services delivery, partial local government participation, or delegated full operational responsibility for local health units.

• Regarding state delegation of responsibility to local governments, in general, **the committee finds that the larger the population served by a single multipurpose government, as well as the stronger the history of local control, the more realistic the delegation of responsibility becomes: for example, to a large metropolitan city, county, or service district. Two attributes of such a locally responsible system are strongly recommended:**

—**To promote clear accountability, public health responsibility should be delegated to only one unit of government in a locality.** For example, in the case of large cities, public health responsibility should be lodged either in the municipal *or* the county government, but not both.

—**Where sparse population or scarce resources prevail, delegation to regional single-purpose units, such as multicounty health districts, may be appropriate.** In order to be effective, health districts must be linked by formal ties to, and receive resources from, general-purpose governments.

Delegation has the great advantage of fostering true independent local advocacy, ownership, and funding capabilities; greater sensitivity to changing local delivery patterns; and greater responsiveness to community priorities. In general, delegation of responsibility to the local level is the committee's preferred option.

• **The committee recommends that mechanisms be instituted to promote local accountability and assure the maintenance of adequate and equitable levels of service and qualified personnel.** Such mechanisms include:

—performance contracting with the state;
—negotiated local standards (for example, based upon the *Model Standards: A Guide for Community Preventive Health Services;* and
—local public health councils.

• **The committee finds that the need for a clear focal point at the local level is as great as at the state level, and for the same reasons. When the scale of** government activity permits, localities should establish public health councils to report to elected officials on local health needs and on the performance of the local health agency.

Federal

The committee is primarily concerned in directing public attention to states and localities where much of the vital decision-making and work of public health goes on. For this reason, research in connection with this study was conducted largely with states and localities as the focus, and public health practice at the federal level was not reviewed in depth. The committee, however, does note the concerns expressed consistently by state and local public health leadership about the lack of a clearly identified national focal point for the exercise of public health leadership and for the support of the state and local public health systems. The impact at the state and local level of the absence of a clear national public health focal point is reflected in the state of affairs discussed in Chapter 5.

- **The committee recommends that the federal government identify more clearly, in formal structure and actual practice, the specific officials and agencies with primary responsibility for carrying out the federal public health functions recommended.**
- **The committee recommends the establishment of a task force to consider what structure or programmatic changes would be desirable to enhance the federal government's ability to fulfill the public health leadership responsibilities recommended in this report.**

SPECIAL LINKAGES

The committee finds that environmental health and mental health activities are frequently isolated from state and local public health agencies, resulting in disjointed policy development, fragmented service delivery, lack of accountability, and a generally weakened public health effort.

Environmental Health

Many environmental health concerns and the authority to deal with them have been removed from the purview of public health agencies. This has led to diffused patterns of responsibility, lack of coordination, and inadequate analysis of the health effects of environmental problems. As a result, society's ability to deal appropriately with these vital issues has been constrained.

- **The committee recommends that state and local health agencies strengthen their capacities for identification, understanding, and control of environmental problems as health hazards. The agencies cannot simply be**

advocates for the health aspects of environmental issues, but must have direct operational involvement. The agencies should have expertise, particularly at the state level, in environmental health science planning and operations, as well as environmental health risk assessment and management. They should maintain ongoing working relationships with organizations that have access to relevant environmental data, encourage regional cooperation in controlling environmental hazards within the state, and work to establish similar cooperation across state lines. In addition to environmental services traditional to the public health mission, such as outdoor air and drinking water quality, food protection, and control of occupational hazards, public health agencies should concern themselves with toxic exposures, pesticide management, indoor air pollution, the health and safety features of health facilities, and groundwater contamination.

Mental Health

The relationship between public health and mental health has been complex and sometimes counterproductive. Although each field has developed useful scientific knowledge and expertise, the separation of the two fields has often produced fragmentation at the service delivery point to the detriment of clients. The existing interface between core public health disease prevention and health promotion and similar efforts in mental health is inadequate to fulfill either the public health mission or the mission of mental health.

● **The committee recommends that those engaged in knowledge development and policy planning in public health and in mental health, respectively, devote specific effort to strengthening linkages with the other field, particularly in order to identify strategies to integrate these functions at the service delivery level.**

● **The committee recommends that a study of the public health/mental health interface be done in order to document how the lack of linkages with public health hampers the mental health mission.**

In contrast to environmental health and mental health, where the problem is isolation from and lack of coordination with public health, the committee believes that social services and indigent medical care are often inappropriately linked organizationally with core public health services, so that public health functions are impaired.

Social Services

In many states and some localities, public health functions are subsumed organizationally under a "super" department of human services (see Appendix A). It is important to develop and sustain productive interactions between activities aimed primarily at improving health and social services directed at general improvements in the quality of life. Examples of areas that benefit from these interactions are maternal and child health and substance abuse. In many such departments, however, the emphasis on the welfare payment role, on certifying client eligibility to receive income maintenance, and on making the payment creates a negative image and detracts from organized community effort to maintain crucial public health functions as well as from the delivery of substantive social services. Desirable integration of service delivery at the client level does not mean that organization and policy must be unified.

• **The committee recommends that public health be separated organizationally from income maintenance, but that public health agencies maintain close working relationships with social service agencies in order to act as effective advocates for, and to cooperate with, social service agency provision of social services that have an impact on health.**

Care of the Medically Indigent

Many state and local health agencies have become providers of last resort for uninsured persons and Medicaid clients unable to secure services in the private sector. This development is consistent with the committee's belief that government is obliged to assure all members of society access to services and to guarantee a basic set. But the responsibility for providing medical care to individuals—precisely because it is so compelling—has drained vital resources and attention away from disease prevention and health promotion efforts that benefit the entire community. These latter efforts encounter great difficulty in competing for policy attention with personal health services. The U.S. failure to find a societywide answer to the question of financial access to needed care has seriously strained the public health system.

• **The committee endorses the conclusion of the President's Commission for the Study of Ethical Problems in Medical Care and Biomedical and Behavioral Research, that:**

Society has an ethical obligation to ensure equitable access to health care for all. . . . The societal obligation is balanced by individual obligations . . . to pay a fair share of the cost of their own health care and take reasonable steps to provide for such care when they can do so without excessive burdens. Nevertheless, the origins of health needs are too complex, and their manifestation too acute and severe, to permit care to be regularly denied on the grounds that individuals are solely responsible for their own health. . . . When equity occurs through the operation of private forces, there is no need for government involvement, but the ultimate responsibility for ensuring that society's obligation is met, through a combination of public and private sector arrangements, rests with the Federal government. (President's Commission for the Study of Ethical Problems in Medicine and Biomedical and Behavioral Research, 1983)

• **The committee finds that, until adequate federal action is forthcoming, public health agencies must continue to serve, with quality and respect and to the best of their ability, the priority personal health care needs of uninsured, underinsured, and Medicaid clients.** Nevertheless, Americans should not assume, as they now appear to, that the public health system is adequately equipped to handle these needs, and they should be aware that this responsibility will remain a continuing threat to the maintenance of crucial disease prevention and health promotion efforts.

The committee also wishes to note that even when the problem of financing personal medical care for all Americans is solved, the public health system will and should retain important responsibilities for furnishing specialized personal health services.

Public health personnel are specialists in health problem identification, disease and disability prevention, and health promotion, a multidisciplinary expertise that addresses social and health needs not met simply by financing medical services. The exemplar of this role is the public health nurse engaged in outreach and case finding, direct service delivery, and management of the needs of multiproblem clients. Social workers functioning as case managers can also serve aspects of this role.

STRATEGIES FOR CAPACITY BUILDING

In the effort to equip public health agencies to fulfill adequately their assessment, policy development, and assurance functions, it is necessary to go beyond reorganization to consider how to build agency competence, especially the human resources and skills that will be required for effective action. There are five types of competence needed to improve the ability of public agencies to meet their responsibilities for the people's health: technical, political, managerial, programmatic, and fiscal. Each requires particular strategies and approaches for improvement.

Technical

Public health agencies must be able to acquire and mobilize scientific and other substantive knowledge, data, and technical skills to solve health problems. Currently, technical capacity is unevenly distributed: some states and localities have considerable expertise, others appear deficient. Some regularly publish data, others do not. Some gather data but lack the ability to analyze it adequately.

The committee recommends the following steps to strengthen public health agency technical capacity:

• **A uniform national data set should be established that will permit valid comparison of local and state health data with those of the nation and of other** states and localities and that will facilitate progress toward national health objectives and implementation of *Model Standards: A Guide for Community Preventive Health Services.*

• An institutional home in each state and at the federal level for development and dissemination of knowledge, including research and the provision of technical assistance to lower levels of government and to academic institutions and voluntary organizations.

• Research at the federal, state, and local levels into population-based health problems, including biological, environmental, and behavioral issues. In addition to conducting research directly, the federal government should support research by states, localities, universities, and the private sector.

Political

Public health agencies should be able to mobilize the support of important constituencies, including the general public, to compete successfully for scarce resources, to handle conflict over policy priorities and choices, to establish linkages with other organizations, and to develop a positive public image. The committee's research suggests that public health agencies are having difficulty striking a balance between political responsiveness and professional values. Some endeavor to insulate themselves from politics; others are buffeted by political firestorms. Too frequently, public health professionals view politics as a contaminant rather than as a central attribute of democratic governance.

The committee recommends the following steps to improve political capacity:

• Public health agency leaders should develop relationships with and educate legislators and other public officials on community health needs, on public health issues, and on the rationale for strategies advocated and pursued by the health department. These relationships should be cultivated on an ongoing basis rather than being neglected until a crisis develops.

• Agencies should strengthen the competence of agency personnel in community relations and citizen participation techniques and develop procedures to build citizen participation into program implementation.

• Agencies should develop and cultivate relationships with physicians and other private sector representatives. Physicians and other health professionals are important instruments of public health by virtue of such activities as counseling patients on health promotion and providing immunizations. They are important determinants of public attitudes and of the image of public health. Public health leaders should take the initiative to seek working relationships and support among local, state, and national medical and other professional societies and academic medical centers.

• Agencies should seek stronger relationships and common cause with other professional and citizen groups pursuing interests with health implications, including voluntary health organizations, groups concerned with improving social services or the environment, and groups concerned with economic development.

• Agencies should undertake education of the public on community health needs and public health policy issues.

• Agencies should review the quality of "street-level" contacts between department employees and clients, and where necessary conduct in-service training to ensure that members of the public are treated with cordiality and respect.

Managerial

Public health agencies must have the capacity for organizational planning; development and implementation of programs; deployment of available resources for maximum efficiency and efficacy; leadership, motivation, and development of individual employees; and organizational evaluation and change in response to changes in the agency environment and its social milieu.

Although many public health managers display these capabilities, the emphasis in the field on technical competence and professionalism sometimes leads to a neglect of management as a skill in its own right. Management is often assumed to be purely a matter of common sense or innate ability rather than a body of knowledge that can be acquired through training and experience.

The committee recommends the following measures to strengthen managerial capacity:

• Greater emphasis in public health curricula should be placed on managerial and leadership skills, such as the ability to communicate important agency values to employees and enlist their commitment; to sense and deal with important changes in the environment; to plan, mobilize, and use resources effectively; and to relate the operation of the agency to its larger community role.

• Demonstrated management competence as well as technical/professional skills as a requirement for upper-level management posts.

• Salaries and benefits should be improved for health department managers, especially health officers, and systems should be instituted so that they can carry retirement benefits with them when they move among different levels and jurisdictions of government.

Programmatic

Public health agencies must have the capacity to deal with the "social environment" in fashioning and implementing public health strategies to address behavior-related health problems.

• **The committee recommends that public health professionals place more emphasis on factors that influence health-related behavior and develop comprehensive strategies that take these factors into account.** Broadening public health emphasis from focus on the individual to consideration of the external factors that influence individual behavior can often result in more cost-effective strategies and, in some cases, stronger legal and political support. Public health leadership should consider all of the social, political, economic, psychological, cultural, and physical factors that shape health-related conduct.

Fiscal

Public health agencies must have the capacity to generate enough resources to fulfill statutory responsibilities and established objectives and to use available resources efficiently and effectively. Currently, however, public health functions are handicapped by reductions in federal support; economic problems in particular states and localities; the appearance of new, expensive problems like AIDS and toxic waste; and the diversion of resources from communitywide maintenance functions to individual patient care.

• **The committee recommends the following policies with respect to intergovernmental strategies for strengthening the fiscal base of public health:**

—**Federal support of state-level health programs should help balance disparities in revenue-generating capacities and encourage state attention to national health objectives. Particular vehicles for such support should include "core" funding with appropriate accountability mechanisms, as well as funds targeted for specific uses.**

—**State support of local-level health services should balance local revenue-generating disparity, establish local capacity to provide minimum levels of service, and encourage local attention to state health objectives; support should include "core" funding. State funds could be furnished with strings attached and sanctions available for noncompliance, and/or general support could be provided with appropriate accountability requirements built in. States have the obligation in either case to monitor local use of state funds.**

EDUCATION FOR PUBLIC HEALTH

As a large, complex, socially important service enterprise, public health depends for its effectiveness on well-qualified professionals (Chapter 5). Many educational paths can lead to careers in public health. However, the most direct route, especially for positions of public health leadership, is to obtain a degree from a school of public health.

Training for public health professional work in the field, especially for technical and administrative leadership, now requires greater emphasis in schools of public health. That training involves substantial development in one or more specific aspects of public health, for example, epidemiology, biostatistics, management of personal health services, environmental science, or health education. It also entails an understanding of how a particular discipline relates to the whole of public health, and an appreciation of the relationship of public health to social endeavor as a whole. Public health professionalism further requires commitment to the public good, the value system that gives public health its coherence. Also, public health professionals require an ability to analyze public health problems from the perspective of their particular discipline as these problems emerge over a professional career and an appreciation for and skill in the political process.

The task now is to assist the schools in developing a greater emphasis on public health practice and to equip them to train personnel with the breadth of knowledge that matches the scope of public health.

The task also includes ensuring that public health educational efforts include short courses to upgrade that substantial majority of public health professionals who have not received appropriate formal training, as well as ensuring that public health personnel are abreast of new knowledge and techniques.

To that end the committee recommends that:

• **Schools of public health should establish firm practice links with state and/or local public health agencies so that significantly more faculty members may undertake professional responsibilities in these agencies, conduct research there, and train students in such practice situations. Recruitment of faculty and admission of students should give appropriate weight to prior public health experience as well as to academic qualifications.**

• **Schools of public health should fulfill their potential role as significant resources to government at all levels in the development of public health policy.**

• **Schools of public health should provide students an opportunity to learn the entire scope of public health practice, including environmental, educational, and personal health approaches to the solution of public health problems; the basic epidemiological and biostatistical techniques for analysis of** those problems; and the political and management skills needed for leadership in public health.

- **Research in schools of public health should range from basic research in fields related to public health, through applied research and development, to program evaluation and implementation research.** The unique research mission of the schools of public health is to select research opportunities on the basis of their likely relevance to the solution of real public health problems and to test such applications in real-life settings.

- **Schools of public health should take maximum advantage of training resources in their universities, for example, faculty and courses in schools of business administration, and departments of physical, biological, and social sciences.** The hazards of developing independent faculty resources isolated from the main disciplinary departments on the campus are real, and links between faculty in schools of public health and their parent disciplines should be sought and maintained.

- Because large numbers of persons being educated in other parts of the university will assume responsibilities in life that impact significantly on the public's health, e.g., involvement in production of hazardous goods or the enactment and enforcement of public health laws, **schools of public health should extend their expertise to advise and assist with the health content of the educational programs of other schools and departments of the university.**

- In view of the large numbers of personnel now engaged in public health without adequate preparation for their positions, **the schools of public health should undertake an expanded program of short courses to help upgrade the competence of these personnel. In addition, short course offerings should provide opportunities for previously trained public health professionals, especially health officers, to keep up with advances in knowledge and practice.**

- Because the schools of public health are not, and probably should not try to be, able to train the vast numbers of personnel needed for public health work, **the schools of public health should encourage and assist other institutions to prepare appropriate, qualified public health personnel for positions in the field. When educational institutions other than schools of public health undertake to train personnel for work in the field, careful attention to the scope and capacity of the educational program is essential.** This may be achieved in part by links with nearby schools of public health.

- **Schools of public health should strengthen their response to the needs for qualified personnel for important, but often neglected, aspects of public health such as the health of minority groups and international health.**

- **Schools of public health should help develop, or offer directly in their own universities, effective courses that expose undergraduates to concepts, history, current context, and techniques of public health to assist in the recruitment of able future leaders into the field.** The committee did not conclude whether undergraduate degrees in public health are useful.

- **Education programs for public health professionals should be informed by comprehensive and current data on public health personnel and their employment opportunities and needs.**

CONCLUDING REMARKS

This report conveys an urgent message to the American people. Public health is a vital function that requires broad public concern and support in order to fulfill society's interest in assuring the conditions in which people can be healthy. History teaches us that organized community effort to prevent disease and promote health is both valuable and effective. Yet public health in the United States has been taken for granted, many public health issues have become inappropriately politicized, and public health responsibilities have become so fragmented that deliberate action is often difficult if not impossible.

Restoring an effective public health system cannot be achieved by public health professionals alone. Americans must concern themselves with whether there are adequate public health services in their communities and must let their elected representatives know of their concern. The specific actions appropriate to strengthen public health will vary from area to area and must blend professional knowledge with community values. The committee intends not to prescribe one best way of rescuing public health, but to urge that readers get involved in their own communities in order to address present dangers, now and for the sake of future generations.

REFERENCES

American Public Health Association, Association of State and Territorial Health Officials, National Association of County Health Officials, U.S. Conference of Local Health Officials, U.S. Department of Health and Human Services, Public Health Service. 1985. *Model Standards: A Guide for Community Preventive Health Services.* American Public Health Association, Washington, D.C.

Gilbert, B., Mary K. Moos, and C. A. Miller. 1982. "State Level Decision-Making for Public Health: The Status of Boards of Health." *Journal of Public Health Policy,* March.

Gossret, D., and C. A. Miller. 1973. "State Boards of Health: Their Numbers and Commitments." *American Journal of Public Health* June 63(6):486–493.

Hughes, Dana, Kay Johnson, Janet Simmons, and Sara Rosenbaum. 1986. *Maternal and Child Health Data Book: The Health of America's Children.* Children's Defense Fund, Washington, D.C.

President's Commission for the Study of Ethical Problems in Medicine and Biomedical and Behavioral Research. 1983. *Securing Access to Care.* Government Printing Office, Washington, D.C.

U.S. Department of Commerce, Bureau of the Census. 1986. *Statistical Abstract of the United States,* 106th ed. Government Printing Office, Washington, D.C.

Supplementary Statements

HARVEY I. SLOANE

There is overwhelming evidence from this report, and from a myriad of studies, that the financial problems confronting the poor must be solved before we can have a significant impact on the other health issues confronting the American people.

In describing the crisis of AIDS, teenage pregnancy and Alzheimer's disease, I cannot help but be greatly disturbed by the fact that these are minuscule in proportion to the numbers of people in this country who do not have adequate health care. More importantly, most of the other recommendations in the report to improve our public health system can never be completely implemented without addressing the indigent care problem.

This most commendable report, in my estimation, is severely flawed if it does not come forth with a great sense of urgency to meet the health needs of the 43 million uninsured and underinsured people of this nation. I would ask for the first priority in the recommendations to be a call for the public and private sectors, at the initiative of the federal government, to implement a program that would provide a financing mechanism for the medically indigent in this country. Until we resolve this issue, general public health measures will be secondary.

Most of the industrialized nations of the world have answered the call for insuring health care to the indigent. This report must issue a clarion call for that same action.

ROBERT J. RUBIN

After examining a great deal of information and hearing from numerous witnesses, the committee concluded that the primary public sector responsibility for health rests with the states. I strongly support that belief. The genius of our federal system, however, is that the various states be free to carry out their responsibility in ways that they deem appropriate.

I do not therefore believe that there is one correct structure of state government that will lead to the answer of the public health dilemma so forcefully articulated in this report. Indeed, our own case studies document that many approaches will yield an acceptable solution. Therefore I cannot support a prescriptive approach that seeks to impose a uniform structure on a diverse group of states. This is particularly true as several of the committee's recommendations do not appear to be based on solid evidence, either empirical or practical.

As regards the federal government's role, I believe that the committee did not heed its own words that "reorganizing is frequently the first resort . . . when in many cases the problem is not truly structural." The federal government is *structured* in a way that allows "a clearly defined national focal point for public health leadership." Whether that leadership is exercised appropriately is more frequently a political perception than an empiric finding.

In conclusion, our report has much to commend it to all Americans concerned about the future of our nation's public health. I believe its operational recommendations, however, should have reflected the breadth and diversity that exist among our states as they strive to assure their public's health.

APPENDIXES

A

A Summary of the Public Health System in the United States

PUBLIC HEALTH AGENCIES

This section summarizes the organization of health agencies, the range of activities carried out by them, and their use and allocation of resources at the federal, state, and local levels. When possible, the range of activities of health agencies are categorized by the functions of public health as outlined in Chapter 2: assessment, policy development and leadership, and assurance of access to environmental, educational, and personal health services.

FEDERAL

The federal government plays a large role in the public health system in the country. It surveys the population's health status and health needs, sets policies and standards, passes laws and regulations, supports biomedical and health services research, helps finance and sometimes delivers personal health services, provides technical assistance and resources to state and local health systems, provides protection against international health threats, and supports international efforts toward global health. The federal government does all of these mainly through two delegated powers: the power to regulate interstate commerce and the power to tax and spend for the general welfare. The federal government's regulatory activities, such as labeling hazardous substances, are based in the power to regulate interstate commerce. Its service-oriented programs, such as the cleanup of hazardous substances or financing personal health services through Medicaid and Medicare programs, are based in its power to tax and spend for the general welfare. (Grad, 1981)

At present, the main federal unit with responsibility for public health is the United States Public Health Service in the Department of Health and Human Services. The second major unit is the Health Care Financing Administration, also in the Department of Health and Human Services. Other federal departments also have agencies with responsibilities for health, such as the Food and Nutrition Service in the Department of Agriculture, the Office of Special Education and Rehabilitative Services of the Department of Education, and the Environmental Protection Agency. Their participation will be discussed in a later section of this chapter.

Leadership

The Secretary of the Department of Health and Human Services is chosen by the President of the United States and sits in his Cabinet. The head of the Public Health Service, the Assistant Secretary for Health, is also appointed by the President. The Surgeon General, who is also appointed by the President, acts as an adviser to the Secretary and the Assistant Secretary.

Organization

The United States Public Health Service includes the (1) Centers for Disease Control; (2) the National Institutes of Health; (3) the Food and Drug Administration; (4) the Health Resources and Services Administration; (5) the Alcohol, Drug Abuse, and Mental Health Administration; and (6) the Agency for Toxic Substances and Disease Registry (Figure A.1). Additionally, several offices relating directly to the Assistant Secretary for Health deal with public health issues, such as the Office of Health Promotion and Disease Prevention and the Office of Planning and Evaluation. These offices are concerned with management; health policy, research, and statistics; planning and evaluation; intergovernmental affairs; health promotion; and other special concerns. (Hanlon and Pickett, 1984)

The Centers for Disease Control, the main assessment and epidemiologic unit for the nation, directly serves the population as well as providing technical assistance to states and localities. The National Center for Health Statistics within the Centers for Disease Control is the main authority for collecting, analyzing, and disseminating health data. The Agency for Toxic Substances and Disease Registry, also an assessment unit, focuses on environmentally related diseases. The National Institutes of Health, the primary research arm of the government, both conducts research and supports research projects across the nation. The Food and Drug Administration directly tests and assesses safety of food, drugs, and a wide variety of consumer goods and sets standards for safe use of these items. The Health Resources and Services Administration is primarily concerned with re-

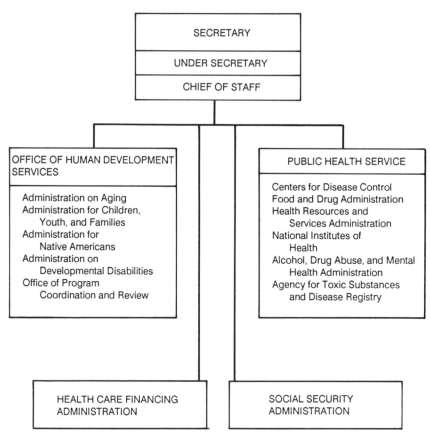

FIGURE A.1 Department of Health and Human Services organization chart.

sources development and health manpower. The Alcohol, Drug Abuse, and Mental Health Administration concentrates on developing programs and setting standards in these areas. Both the Health Resources and Services Administration and the Alcohol, Drug Abuse, and Mental Health Administration establish and support health services through grants and contracts to state and local government agencies, private health care institutions, and individuals. They also act as coordinators and technical assistants to recipients of contracts and grants. Sometimes these agencies provide services, such as the Indian Health Service in the Health Resources and Services Administration, through which the government provides health care services to Native Americans and Eskimos. (Hanlon and Pickett, 1984)

The other major division of the Department of Health and Human Services concerned with public health activities is the Health Care Financing Administration, which operates the Medicare and Medicaid programs. The federal government directly finances health services for elderly Americans through the Medicare program and provides grants to the states through the Medicaid program to assist them in financing health services for poor Americans. A large portion of Medicaid money also goes to finance long-term care for the elderly.

Other operating divisions of the Department of Health and Human Services are primarily oriented toward human and social services. These offices, although not designated specifically for health, conduct many health-related activities. For example, the Office of Human Development Services houses the Administration on Aging and the Administration on Developmental Disabilities, both of which are involved in long-term health care issues. (Figure A.1; Hanlon and Pickett, 1984)

The Department of Health and Human Services also operates regional offices in Boston, New York, Philadelphia, Atlanta, Chicago, Dallas, Kansas City, Denver, San Francisco, and Seattle, which are involved in program development and provide technical assistance to states and local areas within their region. They also oversee programs contracted from the federal government to the states.

Activities

The federal government is involved in each of the public health functions outlined in Chapter 2. The examples of each type of activity are numerous and occur throughout the branches of the Public Health Service and the Health Care Financing Administration, as well as in related government agencies. For example, assessment is a major responsibility of the Centers for Disease Control and the National Center for Health Statistics, but also takes place in the Health Resources Administration, which collects data on health manpower; the Food and Drug Administration, which inspects foods, drugs, and other products; the Office of Disease Prevention and Health Promotion, which collects statistics on prevention activities and the population's health status; the National Institute of Mental Health, which collects data on inpatient and outpatient mental health services; and the Health Care Financing Administration, which collects information on use of health services. Biological research is mainly the task of the National Institutes of Health, and epidemiologic research is mainly the task of the Centers for Disease Control.

The National Center for Health Services Research, under the Office of the Assistant Secretary for Health, is the main authority for policy and health services research. But policy research and health services research can be sponsored by any of the many offices. The Health Care Financing Administration, for example, has an office of research and development. Policy-setting and providing technical assistance take place in nearly all federally conducted programs.

Financing personal and public health services is mainly the task of the Health Care Financing Administration's Medicare and Medicaid offices, but grants for specific services are administered throughout the Department of Health and Human Services. Personal health services are directly delivered by the federal government under the auspices of the Health Resources and Services Administration in the Indian Health Service, but also by the Veteran's Administration and the Department of Defense in military clinics and hospitals.

Overall, federal activities fall into two major categories: those that are conducted directly by the federal government—assessment, policy-making, resources development, knowledge transfer, financing, and some delivery of personal health care—and those that are contracted by the federal government to states, localities, and private organizations—the majority of direct service programs. (Hanlon and Pickett, 1984)

The major portion of the federal government's health business is conducted through contracts and grants to states, localities, and private providers and organizations. The federal government acts through financing intergovernmental and interorganizational contracts to encourage various public health initiatives, convening participants around an issue, coordinating activities, and developing state and local provider contracts. In return for federal funds, states, localities, and private organizations must follow the federal standards and policies set in the contract. Thus in many programs, the federal government takes an oversight, policy-setting, and technical assistance role, rather than a direct provider role. Federal contracts can take the form of seed money for researching and developing new programs, such as Community Mental Health Centers, or they can be support for ongoing activities, such as the Early Periodic Screening, Detection, and Treatment Program. Contracts can be made with agencies to operate specific public health programs or to support general agency activities. Contracts can also be made with health care providers, such as nursing homes or home health agencies, for directly delivering personal health services. Contracts with local areas and providers may be operated through the states or be made directly with the local areas and private sector.

Most contracts to states and localities were initially offered as "categorical" grants, focusing on particular health issues or populations, for example, research training grants for education, nutrition information programs, substance abuse and mental health programs, and family planning programs. In the early 1980s, the federal administration grouped numerous categorical grants to states into four major "block" grants: one in preventive health, one in maternal and child health, one in primary care, and one in alcohol, drug abuse, and mental health. However, a number of categorical aid programs remain, both as grants to states and localities and to private providers. (Hanlon and Pickett, 1984)

Resources

In 1986, the budget for the Public Health Service totaled about $10 billion and is projected to exceed $12 billion by 1988. The budget of the Department of Health and Human Services was $353 billion in 1986. (This figure includes the Public Health Service budget.) A large portion of the department's budget, more than $197 billion, was allotted for the Social Security Program. Another large portion, about $95 billion, was allotted to the Health Care Financing Administration for the Medicare and Medicaid programs. (Executive Office of the President, Office of Management and Budget, 1987) In 1984, about $1 billion of the total departmental budget was spent in contracts to state health agencies; another half billion was contracted directly to local areas for health programs. (See Figures A.2 and A.3; Public Health Foundation, 1984)

To put federal health spending in perspective, the Health Care Financing Administration reports that *federal* expenditures in health were $112 billion in 1984; *public* expenditures (all government) in health care were $160

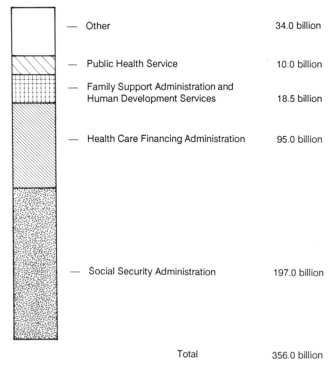

— Other		34.0 billion
— Public Health Service		10.0 billion
— Family Support Administration and Human Development Services		18.5 billion
— Health Care Financing Administration		95.0 billion
— Social Security Administration		197.0 billion
Total		356.0 billion

FIGURE A.2 Expenditures of the Department of Health and Human Services, 1986. SOURCE: Office of Management and Budget, 1987.

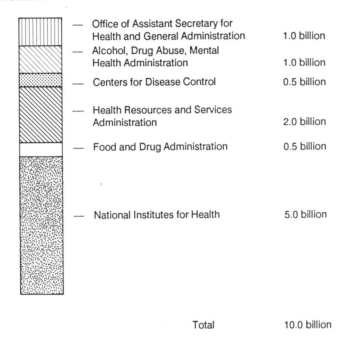

—	Office of Assistant Secretary for Health and General Administration	1.0 billion
—	Alcohol, Drug Abuse, Mental Health Administration	1.0 billion
—	Centers for Disease Control	0.5 billion
—	Health Resources and Services Administration	2.0 billion
—	Food and Drug Administration	0.5 billion
—	National Institutes for Health	5.0 billion
	Total	10.0 billion

FIGURE A.3 Expenditures of U.S. Public Health Service, 1986. SOURCE: Office of Management and Budget, 1987.

billion; and *national* health expenditures (including both public expenditures and private funds for health care and medical care) were in the range of $387 billion. (Bureau of Data Management and Strategy, Health Care Financing Administration, 1985) *Federal* expenditures per person were about $460 (U.S. Department of Commerce, 1986), and *national* health expenditures per person were $1,580. (Bureau of Data Management and Strategy, Health Care Financing Administration, U.S. Department of Health and Human Services, 1985)

Federal spending in health and national spending on health have been subjects of great controversy in the 1980s. Federal spending on health increased dramatically between the 1960s and 1980s, to the extent of several hundred percent in some programs. (Bureau of Data Management and Strategy, Health Care Financing Administration, U.S. Department of Health and Human Services, 1985) Many new programs were also initiated in the 1960s. Cutbacks in federal health spending have been a major goal of the federal administration in the 1980s. For example, the block grants initiated in 1981 included a 25 percent cut in funding to states for the categorical programs included. (Omenn, 1982) (A portion of price cutbacks have since been restored.) Remaining categorical grants were also cut back.

Although federal spending in health continues to increase, it is doing so at a slower pace (U.S. Department of Commerce, 1986)

In terms of personnel, more than 128,000 people are employed by the Department of Health and Human Services. Numerous others are employed in health-related positions in other agencies such as the Department of the Interior and the Environmental Protection Agency.

STATE

States are the principal governmental entity responsible for protecting the public's health in the United States. They conduct a wide range of activities in health. State health agencies collect and analyze information; conduct inspections; plan; set policies and standards; carry out national and state mandates; manage and oversee environmental, educational, and personal health services; and assure access to health care for underserved residents; they are involved in resources development; and they respond to health hazards and crises. (Hanlon and Pickett, 1984; Public Health Foundation, 1986b) States carry out most of their responsibilities through their police power, the power "to enact and enforce laws to protect and promote the health, safety, morals, order, peace, comfort, and general welfare of the people." (Grad, 1981) In the tenth amendment of the U.S. Constitution, states and the people are designated as the repository of all government powers not specifically designated to the federal government. States, as sovereign governments, derive plenary and inherent power to govern from their people. As guardians of the public interest, states have inherent power to act to protect citizens of the state for the good of the entire citizenry. Massachusetts, the first state to establish a State Board of Health, did so "in the interests of health and life among the citizens of the Commonwealth." (Hanlon and Pickett, 1984) States also have the power to delegate agencies with authority to carry out activities in their interest. As phrased in a state law of Virginia,

The General Assembly finds that the protection, improvement and preservation of the public health and of the environment are essential to the general welfare of the citizens of the Commonwealth. For this reason, the State Board of Health and the State Health Commissioner, assisted by the State Department of Health, shall administer and provide a comprehensive program of preventive, curative, restorative, and environmental health services, educate the citizenry in health and environmental matters, develop and implement health resource plans, collect and preserve vital records and health statistics, assist in research, and abate hazards and nuisances to the health and to the environment, both emergency and otherwise, thereby improving the quality of life in the Commonwealth. (Department of Health, Commonwealth of Virginia, 1984)

Leadership

There are 55 state health agencies in the country (the 50 states plus the District of Columbia, Guam, Puerto Rico, American Samoa, and the U.S. Virgin Islands). Each state agency is directed by a health commissioner or secretary of health. Each also has a state health officer, who is the top public sector medical authority in the state. In many states, the state health officer is the director of the state health agency. In some states, the state health officer works for the director, who is an administrator of a larger agency or department. State health officers are appointed either by the governor, the State Board of Health, or an agency head. (Council of State Governments, 1985). Most states require the state health officer to have a degree in medicine, and some require a degree in public health or public health experience. (Table A.1; American Medical Association, Department of State Legislation, 1984) The average term of a state health officer is about 2 years. (Gilbert et al., 1982). The annual salary of state health officers varies substantially among states. In 1986, five states paid more than $80,000 per annum and eight states paid less than $50,000. (Table A.2; Council of State Governments, 1987)

Twenty-four states have boards of health. In general, boards are responsible for policy-making and for spending. The boards' relationships to the health officers vary. In most states, the health officer reports to the board. In some, the health officer is a board member. More than 90 percent of the appointments to boards of health are made by the governor. The remainder are appointed by professional associations or by the state health agency director. About three-quarters of the members of state boards of health are health professionals, and, among these, most are physicians. The average term of a board member is 4 years. (Gilbert et al., 1982)

Organization

State health agencies are organized in one of two models: as a free-standing independent agency responsible directly to the governor or the Board of Health or as a component of a superagency. Of the 55 state agencies, 33 are independent agencies and 22 are divisions of superagencies. (Public Health Foundation, 1986b) In 1980, 34 were independent and 21 were superagencies. (See Table A.3; Association of State and Territorial Health Officials, 1981)

The scope of responsibilities of independent agencies and superagencies varies. Fourteen state health departments are also the main environmental agency in their state; fifteen are the mental health agency; and eleven are also the state Medicaid agency. (Public Health Foundation, 1986b) A few states have changed organizational responsibilities since 1980. (Table A.3; Association of State and Territorial Health Officials, 1981)

TABLE A.1   State Health Officers

	Number of States
A. APPOINTMENT PROCEDURES	(n = 49)
Appointed by Governor	33
Appointed by Agency Director	10
Appointed by State Board of Health	6
	Number of States
B. EDUCATIONAL AND EXPERIENCE REQUIREMENTS	(n = 46)
Medical Degree	25
Medical Degree + Masters of Public Health	8
Medical Degree + Public Health Experience	10
Public Health Experience	3

SOURCES: A. Council of State Governments, 1985; B. American Medical Association, Department of State Legislation, Division of Legislative Activities, 1984.

TABLE A.2   Annual Salaries: Principal State Health Officials, 1986

State or Other Jurisdiction	Annual Salary ($)	State or Other Jurisdiction	Annual Salary ($)
Alabama	96,168	New Hampshire	54,640
Alaska	66,816	New Jersey	70,000
Arizona	63,992	New Mexico	52,260
Arkansas	65,777	New York	85,000
California	78,207	North Carolina	94,380
Colorado	78,450	North Dakota	68,000
Connecticut	66,431	Ohio	68,515
Delaware	60,000	Oklahoma	80,752
Florida	37,000	Oregon	50,304
Georgia	80,250	Pennsylvania	51,500
Hawaii	50,490	Rhode Island	72,347
Idaho	57,033	South Carolina	77,028
Illinois	65,000	South Dakota	43,596
Indiana	47,554	Tennessee	58,500
Iowa	36,400	Texas	66,640
Kansas	N.A.	Utah	77,298
Kentucky	75,300	Vermont	56,992
Louisiana	63,327	Virginia	74,194
Maine	41,240	Washington	78,900
Maryland	68,500	West Virginia	54,500
Massachusetts	54,557	Wisconsin	61,195
Michigan	70,000	Wyoming	55,327
Minnesota	59,774	District of Columbia	65,930
Mississippi	67,290	American Samoa	35,504
Missouri	62,100	Guam	36,838
Montana	35,957	No. Mariana Is.	44,000
Nebraska	59,172	Puerto Rico	40,000
Nevada	43,533	Virgin Islands	43,058

SOURCE: Council of State Governments. 1987.

TABLE A.3   State Health Agency Organization, 1980, 1984

	Number of States	
Organization	1980	1984
A. STRUCTURE		
Superagencies	21	22
Independent	34	33
B. AUTHORITY		
Lead Environmental Agency	16	14
Lead Mental Health Agency	13	15
Lead Medicaid Authority	10	11

SOURCES: Association of State and Territorial Health Officials, National Public Health Program Reporting System, 1981, vol. 1; Public Health Foundation, 1986b, vol. 2.

Organizational units within agencies also vary. Some states have divisions based on regulatory and nonregulatory activities; some have divisions based on different service populations; some have divisions based on different health problems; some have divisions based on environmental and population services. The organizational structure of each state is different and subject to change. (Organizational Charts of State Departments of Health, 1980–1987)

State health agency operations also differ in their level of centralization at the state level. About one-third are completely centralized, operating whatever local health agency units exist in the state. The remainder share operation of programs with local health agencies. Some local health agencies operate completely independently of the state health agency, but in most states state agencies are semicentralized, operating some programs completely, sharing some with locals, and acting as an adviser on some programs. (Miller and Moos, 1981)

Activities

Despite major differences in organization and responsibilities among the state agencies, there are some consistencies in programs handled by the states. For example, nearly all states have programs for vital statistics and in epidemiology. Most conduct planning, and many have planning units. Most have regulatory responsibilities. Almost all states conduct environmental safety programs in sanitation and in water quality. And almost all states are involved in the personal health services. (Public Health Foundation, 1986b)

However, while most states have these programs, the programs can vary in importance and in content. For example, although almost all states have programs for collecting vital statistics, in some states these units report directly to the health officer, and in some the unit may be three or four levels down. While nearly all states collect health statistics, some conduct disease registries and some do not, and some conduct health surveys and some do not. States conduct many similar programs and in some areas offer the same or similar services, but there is also room for tremendous variation in services offered. And there is room for additional unique programs on problems or issues of interest to a particular state. Some state programs are delegated pursuant to federal funding requirements, creating many of the consistencies, and others are state mandated, allowing variation.

Despite differences in program content, the similarities that do exist allow state activities to be generally categorized into the functions of public health outlined in Chapter 2, if it is kept in mind that the activities within these functions do vary.

The best source of data on state health agency activities is the Public Health Foundation, which collects information from states on an annual basis. In the following section, most of the data are taken from the 1986 report of the Public Health Foundation, which reports data from 1984. The data include 46 of the 55 state health agencies. It should be noted that data are necessarily reported according to Public Health Foundation classifications, which follow specific public health activities, rather than functions.

In assessment activities, nearly all the states collect and analyze vital statistics, conduct epidemiology programs, do laboratory analyses, screen the population for health problems, and engage in research. (See Table A.4; Public Health Foundation, 1986b)

Thirty-one states have state centers for health statistics. Twenty-three states report that they have recently completed assessments of their citizens' health as compared to other states. (Office of Disease Prevention and Health Promotion, 1986a) All states screen the population; as a group, they screen for more than 30 types of health problems. All states are involved in communicable disease control, and all but one conduct laboratory analyses. Thirteen states do research and development in their laboratories. (Public Health Foundation, 1986b) Some conduct research on specific health policy issues and health services. For example, many states have established groups to study the problem of providing care to the medically indigent. (Desonia et al., 1985)

Most states reported that they are involved in policy-making and setting standards. Sixteen states have policy analysis and development units. (Organizational Charts of State Health Departments, 1980–1987) Of the 23 states that have conducted health assessments of their populations, 18 are developing goals and objectives based on these assessments. Eight have set up strategic planning and evaluation systems for health assessment. (Office of Disease Prevention and Health Promotion, Public Health Service, U.S. Department of Health and Human Services, 1986a) Thirty states reported involvement in health planning, but nearly all states write plans for specific health services. Thirty-seven states set standards for local health depart-

TABLE A.4   Assessment Activities of State Health Agencies, 1984

	Number of States (*n* = 46)
A. DATA COLLECTION	
Vital Records and Statistics	44
Morbidity	24
Health Facilities	39
Health Manpower	38
Hospital Care	32
Ambulatory Care	19
Long-Term Care	28
Health Systems Funds	22
Health Interview Surveys	20
Health Trends Analyses	35
Population Forecast	31
Disease Registries	8
B. EPIDEMIOLOGY	
Communicable Disease Control	46
Health Screening[a]	46
Vision	39
Nutrition	44
Hearing	40
Hypertension	44
Cervical Cancer	40
Diabetes	34
Sickle Cell Trait	31
Lead Poisoning	27
Speech and Language Disorders	29
Alcohol and Drug Abuse	14
Laboratory Analyses	45
Clinical Services Support	43
Environmental Services Support	40
Toxicologic, Forensic Services Support	35
C. RESEARCH	
Participate in Research Projects	42
Laboratory Research	13

[a]These are selected examples from the more than 30 types of health problems screened by state health agencies.

SOURCE: Public Health Foundation, 1986a, vol. 2.

ments. (Table A.5; American Public Health Association, Health Administration Section, 1984)

In assuring health services, states reported a variety of activities in inspection, licensing, regulation, health education, environmental health, personal health services, and resources development. (See Table A.6) In delivery of health services, individual states may emphasize one type of health service—education, environmental health, or personal health—over another. How-

TABLE A.5 Policy Development Activities of State Health Agencies, 1984

Policy Development	Number of States, 1984 ($n = 46$)
Goals Developed Through Health Assessments of Population	16
Health Planning	30
Categorical Plans	45
Health Services	21
Health Facilities	24
Health Manpower	15
Emergency Medical Services	41
Environmental Health	4
Cancer Prevention and Control	3
Standards for Local Health Agencies	37

SOURCES: Public Health Foundation, 1986b, vol. 2; Office of Disease Prevention and Health Promotion, Public Health Service, U.S. Department of Health and Human Services, 1986.

ever, all of the states report that they conduct some programs in each. Almost all have programs in maternal and child health, communicable disease control, dental health, substance abuse control, public health nursing, nutrition, and services for the mentally retarded.

From the tables, it is easily seen that the activities of any one state agency can differ from another. And, as previously stated, these lists do not indicate the extent of a state's involvement in any one activity. Nor do they indicate states' handling of new responsibilities within an activity. For example, many states have had health education programs for many years, but have increased their efforts in health education in recent years (Office of Disease Prevention and Health Promotion, Public Health Service, U.S. Department of Health and Human Services, 1986a). And 34 states have recently developed special programs or services to assure access to care for the medically indigent, which are not separately catalogued. (Desonia et al., 1985)

Resources

The manner in which states allocate both finances and staff to different activities varies with the programs operated by the state agency, with the size of the state, with balance of responsibilities between states and localities, and with state traditions and priorities. As a group, the 46 state agencies reporting to the Public Health Foundation spent nearly $6 billion for their public health programs in 1984 (Public Health Foundation, 1986b). (This figure was for operation of public health agency programs only, and excludes Medicaid expenditures of states.) The expenditures per state ranged from $646 million in California to $13 million in Wyoming. (California is the most populous state in the country, and Wyoming is the least, save Alaska.) (U.S. Department of Commerce, 1986) Expenditures vary both with size of population and with the scope of responsibilities carried out by state agencies. Public health agency dollars per citizen range from the low 20s to the high 20s between states. (U.S. Department of Commerce, 1986)

In 1984, about 54 percent of the states' total spending was derived from state funds; 37 percent came from federal contracts and grants; 5 percent were from fees and reimbursements; about 2 percent came from local funds; and 2 percent from other sources. Of the federal contract and grant money for states, 1.5 percent was designated for general administration purposes or

TABLE A.6   Assurance Activities of State Health Agencies, 1984

	Number of States ($n = 46$)		Number of States ($n = 46$)
A. INSPECTION		D. ENVIRONMENTAL	
Food and Milk Control	43	Individual Water Supply	
Product Safety,		Safety	35
Substance Control	29	Water Pollution	25
Institutional Safety	37	Sewage Disposal	
Housing, Public		Systems	38
Lodging, Recreational			
Facility Safety	42	E. PERSONAL HEALTH SERVICES	
Health Facility Safety		Ambulatory Services	46
and Quality	41	Maternal and Child	
		Health	46
B. LICENSING		Obstetrical Care	28
Health Services	43	Prenatal Care	46
Health Facilities	41	Family Planning	46
Health Manpower	40	Home Health Care	38
		Immunizations	46
C. HEALTH EDUCATION		Dental Health	46
Health Education	46	Handicapped Children	36
Health Promotion and		Mental Retardation	27
Disease Prevention	31	Mental Health	29
		Alcohol Abuse	24
D. ENVIRONMENTAL		Drug Abuse	20
Air Quality	21	Chronic Disease	45
Occupational Health and		Inpatient Services	
Safety	23	Funded	42
Noise Pollution	15	Inpatient Facilities	
Radiation Control	36	(State-Run)	19
Solid Waste			
Management	22	F. RESOURCES DEVELOPMENT	
Hazardous Waste			
Management	25	Health Services	45
Public Water Supply		Health Facilities	39
Safety	37	Health Manpower	44

SOURCE: Public Health Foundation, 1986a, vol. 2.

"core" support. The remainder was designated for particular categories of health services or "categorical" programs, such as maternal and child health or migrant health. The percentages from each source vary by state. For example, in 3 states more than half the state's expenditures came from federal funding; in 24 states one-quarter to one-half of the state's expenditures came from federal funding; and in 14 states, less than one-quarter of the state's total expenditures was from federal funding. (Table A.7; Public Health Foundation, 1986a,b)

In 1980, the state health agencies spent less than they did in 1984. The 55 reporting to the Public Health Foundation in that year had expenditures of nearly $5 billion. Their sources of funding were about 45 percent from state revenues, 28 percent from federal grants and contracts (which were still categorical at that time and not yet grouped into block grants), 20 percent from local sources, and 7 percent from fees, reimbursement, and other sources. (Table A.7; Association of State and Territorial Health Officials, National Public Health Program Reporting System, 1981)

The increases in state expenditures from 1980 to 1984 do not reflect an increase in buying power. For example, in 1980 the states reported tremendous increases in health spending since 1976, from about $2.5 billion to $4.5 billion. But when the figures were adjusted for inflation using the consumer price index, the real dollar amount reflected an annual 2 percent decrease rather than the seeming annual 15 percent increase. (Association of State and Territorial Health Officials, National Public Health Program Reporting System, 1981) Although inflation rates from 1980 to 1984 were somewhat less than those in the late 1970s, increases in real spending power during this time was still substantially less than that indicated by dollar increases, averaging at about a 2 percent annual increase. (Public Health Foundation, 1987)

It is also important to note that decreases in federal financing are not apparent when percentages of sources of money are considered. Many state

TABLE A.7   Sources of State Health Agency Funds in Percentages, 1980, 1984

Source of Funds	Percentage	
	1980	1984
State	45	54
Federal Contracts and Grants	28	37
Local	20	2
Fees and Reimbursements	7	5
Other	—	2

SOURCES: Public Health Foundation, 1986b, vol. 1; Public Health Foundation, 1981, vol. 1.

TABLE A.8   State Health Agency Areas of
Expenditure in Percentages, 1980, 1984

| | Percentage | |
Areas of Expenditure	1980	1984
Personal Health	74	74
Environmental Health	9	7
Health Resources	7	9
Laboratory	4	3
Administration	6	5

SOURCES: Public Health Foundation, 1986b, vol. 1; Public Health
Foundation, 1981, vol. 1.

programs are funded through formulas specifying proportions of state and
federal funding. During the early 1980s, the federal government cut grants
to states through the block granting process, and only a few states reported
that they intended to make up for the cuts with state funds. Many states
reported that they expected to handle the cuts by reducing expenditures in
programs proportionally to the federal cuts. (O'Kane, 1981) Consequently,
proportions of federal and state financing have remained relatively steady.

In terms of general program content area, in 1984 states spent about 74
percent of their funds on personal health services (including some programs
otherwise categorized above as assessment such as screening, epidemiology,
laboratories, and immunizations), 8 percent on environmental services, 8
percent on health resources, 6 percent on general administration, and 3
percent on laboratories (Public Health Foundation, 1984). These percentages are much the same as those for 1980. (See Table A.8; Association of
State and Territorial Health Officials, National Public Health Program Reporting System, 1981)

Total state expenditures for activities in the functions of public health
defined in Chapter 2 are listed in Table A.9. The majority of state expenditures went to assurance activities, and within that category, personal health
services. Assessment activities were the second greatest expense. (Public
Health Foundation, 1984) Of course, individual state expenditures on any
one activity vary. While total state expenditures on health statistics activities
amounted to $59 million, New Jersey and California spent more than $3
million each on health statistics activities, and Wyoming and Delaware spent
less than 250 thousand each. And Kentucky spent more than $1 million on
health planning, while the majority of states spent nothing. (Public Health
Foundation, 1984)

In staffing, 47 states reported employing a total of 108,100 employees in
1982. The number of employees in each state ranged from a high of 15,100 in
Puerto Rico, to a low of 143 in Idaho. The ratio of health agency staff to

population ranged from 216 employees per 10,000 persons in the Virgin Islands to 0.8 and 0.9 per 10,000 in Illinois, Iowa, and Washington. These wide variations reflect, to a large extent, variations in responsibilities. State health agencies that are also the mental health agencies or the environmental health agencies for their state, or state health agencies that operate institutions, tend to have larger staffs. The mean number of employees for states acting as mental health authorities and/or operating institutions was 3,800, while the mean for agencies not having these responsibilities was 1,100. (Association of State and Territorial Health Officials Foundation, 1985b) (Other states also have employees working in mental health and environmental protection, but they work in other agencies.) About half of the states reported that their staffing figures showed an overall decrease in number of employees during the previous 5 years. Some of the decreases could be attributed to changes in state health agency responsibilities, notably giving up institutions or authority as the mental health agency. Nearly a third of the agencies reported that they had increased staff in the previous 5 years. (Association of State and Territorial Health Officials Foundation, 1985b) Changes since 1982 have not been reported.

TABLE A.9   Totals Amounts of State Health Agency Spending by Function, 1984

Functions of Public Health	Amount ($ millions)
A. ASSESSMENT	
Health Statistics	59
Communicable Disease Control	160
Screening	27
General Epidemiology	45
Laboratory Analysis and Research	17
B. POLICY DEVELOPMENT	
Planning	6
C. ASSURANCE	
Inspections	98
Regulation	107
Health Education	16
Environmental Health	300
Personal Health	4,000
Maternal and Child Health	2,000
Immunizations	38
Inpatient Institutions (State-Run)	900

SOURCE: Public Health Foundation, 1986b, vol. 1.

TABLE A.10 State Agency Staffing by Area
of Specialization, 1982

Area of Specialization	Percentage, 1982	Percentage Change, 1977–1982
Personal Health	64	
Noninstitutional	31	+7.8
State-Run Institutions	33	−11.5
Environmental Health	8	−8.2
Health Resources	8	−2.4
Laboratory	6	−6.9
Administration	8	−1.3
Not Identifiable by Program Area	6	+82.8

SOURCE: Association of State and Territorial Health Officials Foundation, 1985b.

States reported that most of their staff were employed in personal health programs, with half employed in institutions and half employed in non-institutional health programs. Professional, technical, and administrative staff composed 59 percent of the total staff; clerical staff, 41 percent. States reported increases in staff involved in personal health services in the 5 years prior to 1982 and slight decreases in all other areas. (See Tables A.10 and A.11) However, a large increase was shown in staff not reported by program area. (Association of State and Territorial Health Officials Foundation, 1985b) Staff composition of individual agencies, and changes in that composition, of course differ.

It should be kept in mind that state health agency expenditures and staffing are only a small part of the nation's allocation of resources to health. These figures do not include expenditures and staffing of other agencies for health-related programs, nor those of the private providers and organizations.

LOCAL

Local health departments are the "front line" of public health agencies. They are generally responsible for direct delivery of public health services to the population. They conduct communicable disease control programs; provide screening and immunizations; collect health statistics; provide health education services and chronic disease control programs; conduct sanitation, sanitary engineering, and inspection programs; run school health programs; and deliver maternal and child health services, public health nursing services, mental health services, and other home care and

TABLE A.11   State Agency Staffing by Profession, 1982

Profession	Percentage, 1982	Percentage Change, 1977–1982
Professional, Technical,		
Administrative	59.0	
Nurses	20.0	+ 2.4
Engineers and Sanitarians	7.0	− 10.3
Laboratory Technicians	6.0	− 3.4
Physicians	3.0	− 22.5
Dentists	0.5	− 8.6
Health Educators	0.5	− 10.1
Planners, Program Analysts	2.0	+ 49.2
Administrative	5.0	0.0
Nutritionists, Dieticians	1.0	+ 44.0
Social Workers	2.0	− 11.7
Other	12.0	
Clerical and Support Staff	41.0	

SOURCE: Association of State and Territorial Health Officials Foundation, 1985b.

ambulatory care services. (Hanlon and Pickett, 1984; Miller et al., 1977)

Local health departments carry out their activities under authority delegated by their state or by local jurisdictions. State legislatures may delegate power to local agencies to conduct activities in the state interest. In doing so, legislatures may delegate local health departments only to carry out administrative functions of the state, such as enforcing the state public health code, or they may empower city and town governments with regulatory or rule-making powers. "Such a delegation of rule-making powers is, of course, quite common in the public health field, with numerous local legislative bodies—such as city councils and boards of aldermen—and state and local boards of health being authorized to promulgate public health ordinances or health codes, or other species of rules and regulations relating to public health." (Grad, 1981) Local health departments are traditionally viewed as empowered by the state with delegated authority. However, cities and towns may exercise powers autonomously, as chartered by the state, and may empower local health departments. Additionally, under the concept of home rule—the authority of localities to make decisions concerning their own welfare—jurisdictions not incorporated as cities or towns may also assign responsibilities to local health departments. (Grad, 1981) Localities may not, of course, assign responsibilities to local health departments that are in conflict with state laws and regulations. Thirty states allow home rule. (Beyle and Dusenbury, 1982)

Leadership

There are about 3,000 local health departments in the United States. (Miller and Moos, 1981) The number of local health departments in a state ranges from none in Rhode Island, Vermont, Delaware, and the District of Columbia to 159 in Georgia. Each of these departments is either directed by a local health officer or by an administrator, who works in cooperation with the local health officer.

Directors of local health agencies are generally appointed by the leaders of the jurisdiction for which they work, county supervisors, city and town councils, or the mayor. Some local health directors are employees of or appointed by the state health department. In most states, local health department directors are required to have a valid license to practice medicine in the state, but many allow nonphysicians to act as local health directors if they have public health or administrative experience. (See Table A.12) About two-thirds of the local health department directors in the country are physicians, nearly one-third have a master's degree in public health, and about one-tenth have a bachelor's degree or less. (Miller and Moos, 1981; Cameron and Kobylarz, 1980) It can be guessed that about one-third of the local health departments have a local board of health. (Miller et al., 1977)

Organization

Local health departments vary in jurisdiction and authority. Some health departments serve a single county and some serve groups of counties. Some are municipal. And some serve city–county combinations. (See Table A.13) In about a third of the states, local health departments are district offices of

TABLE A.12   Local Health Officers' Educational and Experience Requirements, 1980

Requirements	Number of States
Require Medical Degree	21
Medical Degree Only	7
Medical Degree Plus Public Health Degree or Public Health Experience	14
Require Medical Degree *or* Other Experience	22
(For Other:) Public Health Degree or Experience	19
General Administrative Experience	3
No Requirements	5

SOURCE: Cameron and Kobylarz, 1980.

state health agencies. In another third, local health agencies are responsible to both local government and the state health agency. In the remaining third, local health departments are autonomous, receiving only consultation and advice from the state. (Miller et al., 1977) Some types of local health jurisdiction and authority are more common in one region of the country than another, but the differences do not necessarily follow state lines. A state can have several types of local health departments within its borders or a single type. In many states, such as California and New Jersey, there are a few large autonomous city health departments and many semiautonomous county health departments.

In some areas, there is no local health department. There are about 3,000 county and municipal health departments in the country, but there are 3,040 counties, 39 independent cities, 18,878 municipalities, and 25 city–county consolidations. (Beyle and Dusenbury, 1982) In some areas without local health departments, the population is served directly by the state health department, as it is in most of South Dakota. But in other areas, the population is not served by either a local health department or the state health department, as in the sparsely populated northwest corner of South Dakota. (See Table A.14; Public Health Foundation, 1986b)

Local health departments also differ in organization, size, and the programs they operate. Many are separate agencies, but some are divisions of health and human services agencies. Many are also the local environmental agency, but others share this responsibility with another local agency. Some are district offices of a larger agency, some operate satellite offices of their own. They may serve only a few hundred people, or hundreds of thousands. They may operate a few services or dozens of programs. And they may have a staff of two people or a staff of hundreds.

It should be noted that data on the activities of local health departments are hard to come by. The most specific data are available from a survey conducted in 1974 by the University of North Carolina. The data gathered by this survey have not been replicated in recent years. Data on local health departments are also available from the Public Health Foundation, but these

TABLE A.13   Jurisdictions of Local Health
Agencies by Percentage, 1974

Jurisdiction	Percentage of Local Health Agencies
Single County	48
Multi-County	9
Cities	14
Towns	9
City–County	20

SOURCE: Miller et al., 1977.

TABLE A.14 Population Coverage by Local and State Health Agencies, 1984

	Number of States
A. PERCENTAGE COVERED BY LOCAL HEALTH AGENCY	
90–100	31
50–90	5
10–50	3
<10	0
B. PERCENTAGE COVERED DIRECTLY BY STATE HEALTH AGENCY	
90–100	4
50–90	3
10–50	3
<10	6
C. PERCENTAGE NOT COVERED BY STATE OR LOCAL HEALTH AGENCY	
90–100	0
50–90	0
10–50	1
<10	2

SOURCE: Public Health Foundation, 1986b, vol. 1.

data are only available as reported by the states to the Public Health Foundation. States report data on local activities differently, and some states do not report these data at all.

Local activities vary most significantly by differing local relationships with their state agency. In each program area, some local health departments conduct the program exclusively, some conduct the program in cooperation with the state agency, and some are not at all involved in the program. For example, although all states are involved in communicable disease control, in 10 percent of the states the local health department is solely responsible for the program, in 76 percent states and locals share responsibility for the program, and in 14 percent it is solely a state responsibility. And these relationships can change from program to program. (Miller et al., 1977)

Activities

Despite tremendous variation in services rendered, there are some similarities in local health department programs. Local health departments can be characterized as mainly involved in providing health education, environmental health services, and personal health services and in conducting inspections. Most are also involved in assessment: collecting data and conducting communicable disease control programs and inspections. Some, but few, local health departments are involved in planning, regulating, setting local policies, and conducting research. (Miller et al., 1977; DeFriese et al., 1981) The most common specific activities of local health departments are shown in Table A.15. Of course, the extent of any one local agency's activity in a particular program varies.

Resources

As a group, local health departments spent nearly $2.5 billion in 1984. This figure had increased marginally from $2.4 billion in 1980. (Public Health Foundation, 1986b). In real dollars, this change reflects a reduction in spending power.

Of the $2.5 billion spent in 1984, nearly $1.3 billion was derived from intergovernmental grants from the state, and the remaining came from other sources. Specifically, funds came from state-financed grants and contracts (28 percent); federal grants and contracts, either directly or as passed on by the state (18 percent); local funds (34 percent); fees and reimbursements (11 percent); other sources (2 percent); and unknown sources (6 percent). In 1980, funds were similarly derived. (See Table A.16; Association of State and Territorial Health Officials, National Public Health Program Reporting System, 1981; Public Health Foundation, 1986b) Of course, sources for a particular agency differ from one agency to another. In California, nearly 60 percent of local expenditures are derived from state funds, while in Washing-

TABLE A.15 Activities of Local Health Agencies, 1974

	Local Agencies (%)
A. ASSESSMENT	
Venereal Disease Control	98
Tuberculosis Control	94
Vital Records and Statistics	N/A[a]
B. ASSURANCE	
Environmental Inspections	96
Education	N/A
Personal Health Services	
Maternal and Child Health	89
Family Planning	63
Immunizations	96
School Health	89
Home Care	77
Ambulatory Care	50
Chronic Disease Control	84
Mental Health Care	47
Institutional Care, Chronic	12
Institutional Care, Acute	8

[a]Not available.

SOURCE: Miller et al., 1977; DeFriese et al., 1981.

TABLE A.16   Sources of Local Health Agency Funds
in Percentages, 1980, 1984

| | Percentage | |
Source of Funds	1980	1984
State Grants and Contracts	27	28
Federal Grants and Contracts	17	18
Local	46	34
Fees and Reimbursements	10	11
Other		2
Unknown		2

SOURCES: Public Health Foundation, 1986b, vol. 1; Association of
State and Territorial Health Officials, 1981.

ton, only about 5 percent of local expenditures are derived from state funds.
(Public Health Foundation, 1986b) In about half the states, local health
departments collect fees and in half they do not. (Miller et al., 1977) These
proportions of funding sources can also vary between local health departments within a state. The amount of money available to individual local
health departments also varies tremendously. Some are well-funded, while
many are severely financially constrained.

A portion of federal block grant money is passed on by states to local
agencies. In 1984, about 35 percent of all maternal and child health block
grant money was spent by local health departments. The amount of maternal
and child health block grant money allocated from states to locals ranges
from 1 percent in Nevada to 100 percent in California. About 38 percent of
all preventive health services block grant money was spent by local health
departments. The percentage allocated from states to locals varied from 3
percent in Pennsylvania to 100 percent in California. Eight states did not
allocate any block grant money to local departments. (Public Health Foundation, 1986b)

In terms of program area, in 1984, as a group, local health departments
spent 58 percent of their funds on personal health services, including maternal and child health, communicable disease control, dental health, chronic
disease control, and mental health services, to name a few. They spent 12
percent of their total funds on environmental health services, including
sanitation programs, water and air quality, and waste management. No
figure is available for spending on health education as a separate program. In
assessment and in policy-setting, local health departments spent 9 percent of
their total funds on health resources, including statistics, planning, and
regulation, and 2 percent of the total on laboratory services. In addition, 6
percent was spent for general administration, and 14 percent was not allocated to program areas. About 2.7 percent of state funds to local health

departments supported general administration activities. In 1980, local spending was similar, but somewhat more was spent on personal health and less on health resources. (See Table A.17; Public Health Foundation, 1986b) Again, these proportions vary from state to state, and within states. In 1984, in Mississippi about 90 percent of local expenditures went for personal health services, while in California only about 10 percent of the total was spent on personal health services. (Public Health Foundation, 1986b)

In general, about a third of the staff of local health departments are administrative or support personnel, about a third are registered nurses, and the other third are sanitarians. There is an average of one physician for every 30 local health department employees. The mean number of employees in a local health department is 34. (Miller et al., 1977) However, the number of staff in a local health department can range from more than 1,000 to just a few. A few local health departments in New Jersey employ two people, contract with a neighboring county for a health officer, and serve about 200 people. Some local health departments are larger than other state health departments. The San Diego health department employs more than 500 people and is responsible for an area the size of Connecticut. The number of physicians in a local health department ranges from one part-time health officer to several full-time staff.

In rating the importance of different factors on their ability to operate programs in 1974, local health departments rated constraints in resources—lack of funds and lack of staff—as the most important. (DeFriese et al., 1981) Since then, resource constraints have not improved for most local health departments. Federal cutbacks incorporated into block grants have, in many cases, been passed on to localities by the states. (O'Kane, 1981) And many states have faced their own fiscal crises in the early 1980s.

TABLE A.17   Local Health Agency Areas of
Expenditure in Percentages, 1980, 1984

Area of Expenditure	Percentage	
	1980	1984
Personal Health Services	76	58
Environmental Services	13	12
Health Resources	3	9
Laboratory	3	2
General Administration	5	6
Not Allocated to Program Area		14

SOURCES: Association of State and Territorial Health Officials, 1981; Public Health Foundation, 1986b, vol. 1.

OTHER PARTICIPANTS IN THE PUBLIC HEALTH SYSTEM

As stated earlier in this chapter, the public health system in the United States is not just composed of the federal Department of Health and Human Services, the state health agencies, and the local health departments. The national public health system includes other representatives within government: congressional committees, state legislature committees, governors' task forces, and county and city officials. It also includes a variety of government agencies dedicated to programs that are closely allied to public health: education agencies, environmental protection and natural resource agencies, mental health agencies, agencies on aging, health financing agencies, social service agencies, agricultural agencies, housing authorities, and traffic and highway agencies. And it includes private sector organizations: professional membership associations, universities, the media, consumer organizations, foundations, private health care providers, the insurance industry, and community clinics. All of these groups can have major influence in the national, state, and local public health systems. They can work with the public health agencies to address health problems—conducting assessment activities, helping set policies, and providing access to personal services. The following section briefly describes the range of actors other than the public health agencies that are important contributors to the public health system. A few representatives of health-related government agencies—those dealing with the environment, mental health and substance abuse, social services and human development, and financing health care—and a few examples of private organizations—professional associations, nonprofit organizations, and consumer groups—are highlighted.

NATIONAL

Governmental

The four congressional committees most involved in health issues include the Senate Labor and Human Resources Committee and the House Interstate and Foreign Commerce Committee, which deal with most health issues, and the Senate Finance Committee and the House Ways and Means Committee, which deal with programs of the Social Security Act. Forty-three other committees and subcommittees work on topics related to health. Examples of the latter include the Senate Committee on Veteran's Affairs and the House Subcommittee on Water Resources of the Committee on Public Works and Transportation. (National Health Council, 1979). Each of these committees and subcommittees develops legislation on different health and health-related issues for the country. Many of the federal policy initiatives carried out by the public health service and others originate with these committees.

In the federal executive branch, numerous agencies other than the Public Health Service conduct health-related activities. These agencies are concerned with the health of special populations or with special problems, including the medical divisions of the army and navy, the Veteran's Administration, the Bureau of Indian Affairs, the Agricultural Extension Service, the Department of Education, the Occupational Health and Safety Administration, the Federal Trade Commission, the Bureau of Labor Standards, the Bureau of Mines, the Maritime Commission, many bureaus within the Department of Agriculture, and the Bureau of Employees' Compensation. Other agencies are concerned with international health interests, including the Agency for International Development and the Department of Defense. (Hanlon and Pickettt, 1984)

In the representative areas of environment, mental health, and social services, there are programs both within the Department of Health and Human Services and outside of that department.

Environmental programs are mainly handled by the Environmental Protection Agency and by the Agricultural Department. These agencies conduct assessment activities, develop policies and standards, provide direct services and technical assistance to states and localities, and conduct research. The Environmental Protection Agency has programs in air pollution and water pollution control, hazardous waste cleanup, control of pesticides, radiation protection, and research. (Haskell and Price, 1973) Some of these programs are direct federal activities, and some provide assistance to state environmental departments and state health agencies. The Agricultural Department has services for food safety and inspection, sanitation, and assessment of both plant and animal diseases. These services are predominantly federally run. The federal government spent more than $3.5 billion on environmental programs in 1986. (Executive Office of the President, Office of Management and Budget, 1987)

The majority of federal mental health programs are sponsored by the Public Health Service in the Alcohol, Drug Abuse, and Mental Health Administration. This administration predominantly conducts its programs through grants and contracts to states, localities, and private organizations. Some additional mental health programs are conducted through other departments, for example, Department of Education programs for the handicapped. The federal government is also involved in directly financing mental health care through the Medicare and Medicaid programs and in directly providing mental health care through the operation of a mental health hospital. The federal government spent more than $3 billion on mental health programs and care in 1983 in contracts and grants and in financing care for individuals. (Mazade et al., 1985a)

Programs devoted to social services and the welfare of citizens are within the Department of Health and Human Services in the Office of Human Development Services and the Family Support Service. These programs are involved in assessment of population needs, policy development, providing technical assistance to the states, and in providing direct services to citizens. Agencies include the Administrations on Aging; Native Americans; Children, Youth and Families; Refugees; and the Developmentally Disabled. Examples of programs in personal health services and social services outside of the Department of Health and Human Services are numerous. The Bureau of Nutrition and Home Economics of the Department of Agriculture works with the agricultural extension service to improve the nutrition of rural populations. The Department of Agriculture also runs the food and nutrition service, including both the food stamp program and the supplemental nutrition program for women, infants, and children. The Department of Defense has hospitals and clinics for military and military dependents. The Veteran's Administration runs hospitals and nursing homes. The Bureau of Mines in the Department of the Interior conducts health, sanitation, and safety programs for employees of the mining industry. The Department of Education promotes programs of health education and health safety, engages in screening and medical examinations of students and teachers, and administers a grant program for vocational education in health. (Hanlon and Pickett, 1984) Some of these programs relate to social service agencies in the states, some to educational departments, and some to health departments. Many provide direct services or assistance to consumers.

Federal spending on personal social and health services is difficult to assess. In 1986 the Office of Human Development Services spent about $5 billion. The Family Support Administration spent about $13 billion. Programs outside the Department of Health and Human Services added considerably to the total spent on personal medical and social services, for example the budget for the Veteran's Administration Medical Care Services was $9 billion in 1986. The Occupational Safety and Health Administration had a budget of $200,000. The budget of the Food and Nutrition Service of the Department of Agriculture was more than $18 billion. The cost of the supplemental nutrition service for women, infants, and children was more than $1.6 billion in 1986. In many states, federally funded nutrition services are the largest public health program. In addition, many personal social and health services are financed by the Health Care Financing Administration and the Social Security Administration, and by programs within the other departments and agencies. In 1986 the Health Care Financing Administration spent more than $70 billion in Medicare expenditures and nearly $25 billion in Medicaid expenditures. That same year the Social Security Administration spent about $10 billion on supplemental security income, which can be used to cover long-term health benefits.

(Executive Office of the President, Office of Management and Budget, 1987)

Nongovernmental

In the private sector, the national organizations with interests in health are almost too numerous to list. There are professional membership organizations for almost every type of health professional and every type of health care organization. Examples include the American Medical Association, the American Nurse's Association, the National Social Workers Association, the American Public Health Association, the National Association of Community Health Centers, the American Hospital Association, and the Association of State Mental Health Agency Directors. Members in these organizations come from both the private and the public sectors. These groups generally serve for members to exchange knowledge and to promote policies. Sometimes they are involved in lobbying Congress for changes in national health policies and regulations, changes in programs, and support for research. For example, the American Medical Association has been active in supporting research related to the health effects of smoking and in antismoking campaigns. The American Public Health Association has taken political positions on nuclear policy and Central American politics, as well as campaign for legislation and education on many health problems such as smoking, teen pregnancy, and injury.

There are also numerous nonprofit associations on the national level that are organized around particular health problems or issues, rather than around a professional discipline. Examples include the American Heart Association, the American Cancer Society, the Alzheimer's Disease and Related Disorders Association, and the American Diabetes Association. These associations also provide arenas for information exchange and policy development, and they sometimes sponsor research in their area of concern. They are also often involved in lobbying for new policies, activities, and the development of resources. For example, the American Cancer Society has been integral in developing resources for cancer research and for promoting antismoking campaigns.

There are also national organizations of citizens focused around health issues or concerned about health in general. Groups include both professionals and consumers and representatives from public agencies and from private providers. Examples include Dissatisfied Parents Together, Alcoholics Anonymous, National Association of Retarded Citizens, National Consumers League, and Gay Men's Health Crisis. These groups are generally involved in information exchange, coalition building, and lobbying. They can be the main force in starting new programs. For example, the Gay Men's Health Crisis has played a central role in starting up community health services for AIDS victims in New York City. The National Association of

Retarded Citizens played a central role in securing resources for community care and health care for mentally retarded citizens across the country.

Finally, at the national level, there are foundations that support health research projects and demonstrations of new health services, including The Robert Wood Johnson Foundation, Pew Memorial Trust, Rockefeller Foundation, Kellogg Foundation, Commonwealth Fund, and The Rosenwald Foundation. They can act much like the federal government in providing grants to local areas for health programs and in supporting research. These foundations can play a strong role in assisting information and policy development, and in providing services in a local area. In 1984, about $10.4 billion were given to health and hospitals in private philanthropy, and about $8 billion were given to social welfare projects. (U.S. Department of Commerce, 1986) A few examples of programs supported by foundations include health care for homeless citizens in 16 cities supported by Pew Memorial Trust, the promulgation of community services for AIDS victims supported by Robert Wood Johnson, and research on access to health care, also by Robert Wood Johnson.

All of these types of private groups can be vital influences in the development of public health policy on the national level and in the carrying out of public health programs, both in national and local settings.

It should be kept in mind that national resources expended on health include the activities of all of these associations and organizations. The nation spent in the range of $387 billion on health and medical care in 1984. (Bureau of Data Management and Strategy, Health Care Financing Administration, U.S. Department of Health and Human Services, 1985) This figure does not, however, include private grants for health services, membership dues, expenditures of agencies other than health agencies, and tremendous amounts of volunteer time. Public health manpower is also present in all of these arenas. There are approximately 62,000 graduates of public health schools and public health programs in this country (Moore and Kennedy, 1987). And there are about 5.6 million health professionals in the country, including about 1.8 million nurses and some 500,000 physicians. (U.S. Department of Commerce, 1986). Some portion of these individuals work in public agencies, many work in medical care, and some work in nonprofit associations. Taken together, they represent the national public health system's workforce.

STATE

Governmental

On the state level, government, public agencies, and private groups are also active in the public health system. Many state legislatures have committees with interests in health issues. And several states have governor-appointed task forces on particular health issues. For example, 22 state legislatures introduced bills concerning access to health care for the medically indigent population in 1984; 20 states organized legislative or gubernatorial study commissions on the issue in 1984. (Desonia and King, 1985) These groups can be the principal public health policymakers in a state. The designation, involvement, and activity of these committees and task forces vary from state to state.

States can have several agencies engaged in activities related to public health, including environmental agencies; social service and welfare agencies; agencies for human development, for aging, and for the developmentally disabled; mental health agencies; Medicaid agencies; education departments; housing authorities; and traffic and highway departments. The exact array of agencies in a given state varies, as does the involvement of the agencies in health issues. In the examples of the environment, social services, and mental health, states have an array of agencies that vary as much as their health agencies. In some states, environmental, social service, and mental health agencies are combined with the state health department, and in some states they are separate agencies. In all states, there are programs in these areas that overlap with those of the health department, regardless of whether the agencies are combined.

A majority of the states have independent environmental agencies. These agencies conduct assessment and address environmental hazards. They can be devoted to single environmental issues—water safety, hazardous waste control, fish and wildlife, air pollution control—or they can be environmental superagencies. Nearly all of the states also have units within their health departments devoted to environmental health concerns, such as sanitation, inspection, water supply, pollution control, and sometimes occupational safety and hazardous materials control; and most state health agencies take the lead responsibility in a state for one or more environmental health services. In some states, these functions are combined. In 11 states, the state health agency is the principal "lead" environmental agency. In 28, another agency fills that function. (In 5 states there is no officially designated lead environmental agency.) In a few of the states in which the health agency is the lead environmental agency, there are additional environmental agencies that coordinate with the health agency. For example, the health department might deal with water supply safety, and a separate agency might deal with toxics and hazardous materials, environmental factors that would affect the water supply. Some states interpret environmental issues as intrinsically related to health, as the cleanliness of the environment directly affects health. Some states interpret environmental activities as conservation of resources. Many states interpret environmental issues as both and separate them between agencies.

In any situation, the activities of environmental agencies and health agencies often overlap. Forty-four state health agencies have lead responsibility for some environmental health programs, even though only 11 are the lead environmental agency. Thirty-two state agencies share responsibility for some environmental programs with another agency, and 26 play a supporting role to another agency that has the lead responsibility for programs. (Public Health Foundation, 1986b; Haskell and Price, 1973)

In 15 states, the state health agency is also the lead mental health agency for the state. (Public Health Foundation, 1986b) In 14 states, the mental health agency is housed within the health and human services superagency; in 5, it is in an independent health agency; in 18, the mental health agency is independent; and in 14, the mental health agency is part of the welfare or social services agency. (National Association of State Mental Health Agencies, 1987). Many states also have separate agencies for developmental disabilities, mental retardation, and substance abuse control.

There can be a good deal of overlap between state health agency concerns and mental health agency concerns. State mental health agencies handle programs of both a public health nature, such as prevention of mental illness, alcoholism and drug abuse prevention, research, and manpower training, as well as personal health services such as treatment of mental illness, rehabilitation for substance abusers, and services for the mentally retarded and developmentally disabled. In 44 states, public health agencies report that they operate programs for the mentally retarded and developmentally disabled; 37 operate mental health programs; 33 have alcohol abuse programs; and 29 have drug abuse programs. (Public Health Foundation, 1986b) All states either operate services for or finance inpatient mental health care. In a few, inpatient mental health, mental disability, and substance abuse services are operated or financed by the state health agency. (Mazade et al., 1985b; Public Health Foundation, 1986b) In each state there is some overlap between public health and public mental health.

In nearly half of the states, the health agency and the social services agency are combined to form superagencies for human services, much like the federal Department of Health and Human Services. These agencies handle social services for the aged; for children, youth, and families; for adolescents; for the developmentally disabled; and sometimes for particular social problems, such as alcoholism and drug abuse—as well as health services for these groups. The remainder of the states have independent social services or welfare agencies. In many states, social services and health services can overlap in areas such as alcohol and drug abuse rehabilitation and mental health or family services and maternal and child health care. Some programs are essentially both social services and personal health services.

Nowhere is the overlap between health and social services more apparent than in the Medicaid program. Many states view Medicaid as a social services program, providing services for disadvantaged citizens. But a few states view Medicaid as a health program, financing health care services. In 14 of the states, the state Medicaid agency is housed within the health and human services superagency. In 27, the Medicaid agency is in an independent welfare or social service agency or in a state welfare agency separate from the health and human services superagency. In 5 states, Medicaid is handled by the independent state health agency, and in 3, Medicaid is a separate agency. (Office of Research and Demonstrations, Health Care Financing Administration, U.S. Department of Health and Human Services, 1983) In any of these cases, there is considerable influence in both directions between public health policy and Medicaid policy. The operation of health programs and the financing of health services are connected, particularly in states in which the state health agency concentrates its efforts on personal health services. In most states, the state Medicaid budget is equal to or far exceeds the public health budget. States spent between $9 million and $370 million on their public health programs in 1980, and between $14 million and $2.7 billion for Medicaid in 1980. (Association of State and Territorial Health Officials, National Public Health Reporting System, 1981; Office of Research and Demonstrations, Health Care Financing Administration, U.S. Department of Health and Human Services, 1983)

Nongovernmental

In the private sector, there are many state-level professional associations, nonprofit associations, and consumer organizations that parallel the national organizations described above. Many are state factions of the national organizations and serve to exchange information, promote policies, and lobby on the state level. There are state medical associations, state nurse's associations, social worker's associations, and public health associations, to name a few.

In addition to state members of national organizations, there are private organizations involved in the public health system that are more visible on the state level. Some states have business coalitions that are involved in health promotion programs at the worksite. The Washington Business Group on Health in Washington, D.C., is an example of this type of organization. Other states have a single major employer that is involved in health promotion. Johnson and Johnson runs a popular "fit for life" program for its employees. Some states have medical schools, public health schools, and nursing schools—Johns Hopkins, Harvard, the University of Washington, the University of California—that are important influences in the public health system in directing policy, providing services, and conducting research. Private health care providers, such as major hospital systems, can also be visible influences in the public health system at the state level. And finally, the media can play a large role in focusing issues and providing information on health at the state level. Many papers, such as *The Washington Post,* have special health sections written for consumers.

LOCAL

Governmental

On the local level, government, local agencies, and private organizations can also be central to the public health system. County supervisors, aldermen (freeholders, selectmen), and mayors can direct the public health system in the same manner that the legislature and the governor direct public health issues and policies on the state level. Local government can also convene task forces and meetings around particular issues.

Local areas can also have other public agencies active in the public health system. All local areas have boards of education, which may be involved in school health and child and adolescent health issues. And they have police and fire departments, which may be active in emergency care.

Local areas may also have agencies involved in environmental protection, social services, and mental health. These agencies vary as significantly from area to area as local health agencies. They can be divisions of the state agencies, or independent. Or they can be district offices. In addition, these agencies can be combined with the health department or separate from the health department, as on the state level. And their organization may parallel state organization, or it may not. Regardless of local organization, environmental, social service, and mental health public agencies have concerns and conduct activities which overlap with those of the local health agency in the same manner that concerns of state agencies overlap. The local health department may monitor an individual's water supply, while a local environmental agency monitors industrial or agricultural water supplies. The local health department may have a substance abuse prevention program, while inpatient mental health services are provided by another agency. And the local health department may provide maternal and child health services to families that go to the welfare agency to apply for Medicaid.

Nongovernmental

Private organizations can also have a powerful influence on a local public health system. In the local arena, the private health care provider becomes particularly visible. In many areas, the physicians working at the local health department, or even the local health officer, may be a private practitioner. Or a private clinic or hospital may be the principal provider of services for a particular area. As on the state and national levels, the media, consumer groups, and professional organizations can also have a major influence on the public health system in a local area. The media, consumers, and professionals can draw attention to issues; they can lobby local government for changes in policy; and they can be sources for information.

CONCLUSION

It should be noted that the public health system, as divided above by national, state, and local settings, is not necessarily that static. There are many channels for information and coordinated activity between national, state, and local levels in both the public and private sectors, just as there is exchange of information and coordination of activity between the health agencies, other agencies, and private actors. The system is both intergovernmental and interorganizational. The amount of interchange and cooperation between government levels and the public and private spheres, however, differs between settings and across issues.

REFERENCES

American Medical Association, Department of State Legislation, Division of Legislative Activities. 1984. *State Health Departments.* American Medical Association, Chicago, Ill.

American Public Health Association, Association of State and Territorial Health Officials, National Association of County Health Officials, U.S. Conference of Local Health Officials, U.S. Department of Health and Human Services, Public Health Service. 1985. *Model Standards: A Guide for Community Preventive Health Services.* American Public Health Association, Washington, D.C.

American Public Health Association, Health Administration Section. 1984. *State Systems of Local Health Department Standards, 1983.* American Public Health Association, Washington, D.C.

Association of State and Territorial Health Officials Foundation. 1984. *Public Health Agencies 1982,* vols. 1, 2, and 4. Association of State and Territorial Health Officials Foundation, Washington, D.C.

Association of State and Territorial Health Officials, National Public Health Program Reporting System. 1981. *Public Health Agencies 1980: A Report on the Expenditures and Activities.* Association of State and Territorial Health Officials, National Public Health Reporting System, Washington, D.C.

Association of State and Territorial Health Officials Foundation. 1985a. *Special Report: Profile of 1983 State Health Agency Data Relevant to the 1990 Objectives for the Nation.* Association of State and Territorial Health Officials Foundation, Washington, D.C.

Association of State and Territorial Health Officials Foundation. 1985b. *Staffs of State Health Agencies.* Association of State and Territorial Health Officials Foundation, Washington, D.C.

Beyle, T., and P. Dusenbury. 1982. "Health and Human Services Block Grants: The State and Local Dimension." *State Government* 55(1):2–13.

Bureau of Data Management and Strategy, Health Care Financing Administration, U.S. Department of Health and Human Services. 1985. *HCFA Statistics.* U.S. Department of Health and Human Services, Washington, D.C.

Cameron, C. M., and A. Kobylarz. 1980. "Nonphysician Directors of Local Health Departments: Results of a National Survey." *Public Health Reports* 95(4):386–397.

Council of State Governments. 1985. *The Book of the States, 1984–5.* Council of State Governments, Lexington, Ky.

Council of State Governments. 1987. *The Book of the States, 1986–87,* vol. 26. Council of State Governments, Lexington, Ky.

DeFriese, G. H., J. S. Hetherington, E. F. Brooks, C. A. Miller, S. C. Jain, F. Kavaler, and J. S. Stein. 1981. "The Program Implications of Administrative Relationships Between Local Health Departments and State and Local Government." *American Journal of Public Health* 71(10):1109–1115

Department of Health, Commonwealth of Virginia. 1984. *The Health Laws of Virginia.* The Mitchie Co., Charlottesville, Va.

Desonia, R., and K. King. 1985. *State Programs of Assistance for the Medically Indigent.* Intergovernmental Health Policy Project, Washington, D.C.

Desonia, R., J. Luehrs, and G. Brown. 1985. *Addressing Health Care for the Indigent: State Initiatives, 1985.* The Intergovernmental Health Policy Project, the National Governor's Association, Washington, D.C.

Executive Office of the President, Office of Management and Budget. 1987. *Budget of the United States Government, Fiscal Year 1988.* Government Printing Office, Washington, D.C.

Gilbert, Benjamin, Merry-K. Moos, and C. Arden Miller. 1982. "State Level Decision Making for Public Health: The Status of Boards of Health." *Journal of Public Health Policy,* March, pp. 51–61.

Gossert, Daniel J., and C. Arden Miller. 1973. "State Boards of Health, Their Members and Commitments." *American Journal of Public Health,* June, 63(6):486–493.

Grad, Frank P. 1981. *Public Health Law Manual: A Handbook on the Legal Aspects of Public Health Administration and Enforcement.* American Public Health Association, Washington, D.C.

Hanlon, G., and J. Pickett. 1984. *Public Health Administration and Practice.* Times Mirror/ Mosby.

Haskell, E., and V. Price. 1973. *State Environmental Management: Case Studies of Nine States.* Praeger Publishers, New York.

Mazade, N., T. Lutterman, and R. Glover. 1985a. *Funding Sources and Expenditures of State Mental Health Agencies: Revenue/Expenditure Study Results Fiscal Year 1983.* National Association of State Mental Health Program Directors, Washington, D.C.

Mazade, N., T. Lutterman, and R. Glover. 1985b. *Selected State and Federal Government Agency Mental Health Expenditures Incurred on Behalf of Mentally Ill Persons.* National Association of State Mental Health Program Directors, Washington, D.C.

Miller, C. A., E. F. Brooks, G. H. DeFriese, B. Gilbert, S. C. Jain, and F. Kavaler. 1977. "A Survey of Local Public Health Departments and Their Directors." *American Journal of Public Health* 67(10):931–939.

Miller, C. A., B. Gilbert, D. G. Warren, E. F. Brooks, G. H. DeFriese, S. C. Jain, and F. Kavaler. 1977. "Statutory Authorizations for the Work of Local Health Departments." *American Journal of Public Health* 67(10):940–945.

Miller, C. Arden, and Merry-K. Moos. 1981. *Local Health Departments: Fifteen Case Studies.* American Public Health Association, Washington, D.C.

Moore, F., and V. Kennedy. 1987. "Analysis of Public Health Workforce." Center for Health and Manpower Policy Studies, University of Texas Health Science Center at Houston, unpublished data prepared for IOM Conference on Education, Training, and the Future of Public Health.

National Association of State Mental Health Agencies, Membership List, 1987.

National Health Council. 1979. *Congress and Health: An Introduction to the Legislative Process and Its Key Participants.* National Health Council, Washington, D.C.

Office of Disease Prevention and Health Promotion, Public Health Service, U.S. Department of Health and Human Services. 1986a. *A Review of State Activities Related to the Public Health Service's Health Promotion and Disease Prevention Objectives for the Nation.* U.S. Department of Health and Human Services, Washington, D.C.

Office of Disease Prevention and Health Promotion, Public Health Service, U.S. Department of Health and Human Services. 1986b. *The 1990 Health Objectives for the Nation: A Midcourse Review.* U.S. Department of Health and Human Services, Washington, D.C.

Office of Research and Demonstrations, Health Care Financing Administration, U.S. Department of Health and Human Services. 1983. *The Medicare and Medicaid Data Book, 1983.* U.S. Department of Health and Human Services, Washington, D.C.

O'Kane, Peggy. 1981. *Survey of Health Block Grant Implementation.* The Intergovernmental Health Policy Project, Washington, D.C.

Omenn, G. S. 1982. "What's Behind Those Block Grants in Health?" *New England Journal of Medicine* 306(17):1057–1060.

Organizational Charts of State Departments of Heath. 1980–1987. Unpublished information collected by the Public Health Foundation for the IOM Committee to Study the Future of Public Health.

Public Health Foundation. 1981. *Public Health Agencies, 1980.* Public Health Foundation, Washington, D.C.

Public Health Foundation. 1986a. *1984 Public Health Chartbook.* The Public Health Foundation, Washington, D.C.

Public Health Foundation. 1986b. *Public Health Agencies 1984,* vols. 1, 2, and 4. The Public Health Foundation, Washington, D.C.

Public Health Foundation. 1987. *Public Health Agencies 1987.* The Public Health Foundation, Washington, D.C.

Public Health Service, U.S. Department of Health and Human Services. 1980. *Promoting Health/Preventing Disease: Objectives for the Nation.* U.S. Department of Health and Human Services, Washington, D.C.

Rabe, Barry G. 1986. *Fragmentation and Integration in State Environmental Management.* The Conservation Foundation, Washington, D.C.

U.S. Department of Commerce. 1986. *National Data Book and Guide to Sources: Statistical Abstract of the United States,* 106th ed. Government Printing Office, Washington, D.C.

U.S. Department of Health and Human Services. 1986. Organizational Chart of the Department of Health and Human Services. U.S. Department of Health and Human Services, Washington, D.C.

Biographies of Committee Members

RICHARD D. REMINGTON, PH.D., is Vice President for Academic Affairs and Dean of the Faculties, University of Iowa Foundation Distinguished Professor of Preventive Medicine and Environmental Health at the University of Iowa. He was named Interim President of the University in July 1987. From 1974 to 1982 he was Dean and Professor at the University of Michigan School of Public Health. For the preceding 5 years he was Associate Dean for Research and Professor of Biometry at the University of Texas School of Public Health at Houston. His interest in public health and statistics has concentrated primarily on the epidemiology and control of cardiovascular diseases and therapeutic clinical trials. He was Vice President for Research and Vice President for Scientific Councils of the American Heart Association and is Past-President of the Association of Schools of Public Health. Among his honors are the Lasker Award, the Gold Heart Award of the American Heart Association and the honorary degree, Doctor of Science, from the University of Montana.

DAVID AXELROD, M.D., has been the Commissioner of Health of New York since January 2, 1979. He joined the staff of the State Health Department in 1968, when he was appointed Director of the Infectious Disease Center in the Division of Laboratories and Research, and assumed the directorship of the Division of Laboratories and Research in 1977. He also served as special assistant to the Commissioner on drinking water pollutants and as a member of several national panels and subcommittees dealing with environmental hazards. From 1962 to 1968, Dr. Axelrod was a commissioned officer in the U.S. Public Health Service, working as a research scientist in the Laboratory of Biology of Viruses at the National Institutes of Health, Washington, D.C. Dr. Axelrod is a research scientist and an authority on environmental toxicology. He was the first to focus state and federal attention on the potential health problems associated with the Love Canal landfill in Niagara Falls and has worked diligently to improve New York State's capability to protect its citizens from environmental health hazards. He has also earned national recognition for his stand on the controversial subject of physician misconduct and discipline and for his innovative health care cost containment initiatives.

EULA BINGHAM, PH.D., is the Vice President for Graduate Studies and Research at the University of Cincinnati and is also a Professor of Environmental Health in the College of Medicine. From 1972 to 1977 she was the Associate Director of the Department of Environmental Health, University of Cincinnati Medical Center, and from 1977 to 1981 held the position of Assistant Secretary of Labor for the Occupational Safety and Health Administration, U.S. Department of Labor. She served as a member of the City of Cincinnati's Board of Health from January 1983 to December 1985. In 1980 she received the Rockefeller Foundation Public Service Award and the Julia Jones Award from the American Lung Association. The American Public Health Association has awarded her both the Homer N. Calvert Award (1980) and the Alice Hamilton Award (1984). She is a member of numerous organizations such as the American Association for Cancer Research, the American College of Toxicology (President, 1981), Sigma Xi, and Collegium Ramazzini. Dr. Bingham is the author of many papers on chemical carcinogenesis, pulmonary toxicology, and public policy issues and serves on many federal, state, and local advisory committees.

JOSEPH BOYLE, M.D., is Executive Vice President of the American Society of Internal Medicine. From 1954 to 1985 he was in the private practice of Internal Medicine and Pulmonology in Los Angeles, Calif. During that time he held an appointment as Associate Clinical Professor of Medicine at the University of Southern California School of Medicine and also served as attending physician in medicine and as a consultant to the Department of Surgery at USC-Los Angeles County Medical Center. He served as consultant to numerous committees and departments for the County of Los Angeles and the State of California. Dr. Boyle has also served as a member of the President's Advisory Council on Environmental Quality and is a former Chairman of the Board of Trustees and Past-President of the American Medical Association; a Past-President of the California Medical Association and Los Angeles County Medical Association; and a Past-President of the California Chapter of the American College of Chest

Physicians. From 1982 to 1987 he was chairman of the Steering Committee for the Health Policy Agenda for the American People.

LESTER BRESLOW, M.D., M.P.H., is Dean Emeritus and Professor, School of Public Health, and Director of Health Services Research, Jonsson Comprehensive Cancer Center, UCLA. Before coming to UCLA, he was with the California State Department of Public Health from 1946 to 1968. He has served as President of the American Public Health Association, of the International Epidemiological Association, and of the Association of Schools of Public Health. In 1959 Dr. Breslow initiated the Human Population Laboratory in Alameda County, Calif. As a member of the Institute of Medicine, he has served on the Council; as founding Chairman, Board on Health Promotion and Disease Prevention; and on several study projects. In 1979 he became the first editor of the *Annual Review of Public Health* and has continued in that capacity. Dr. Breslow has been a frequent consultant to the National Cancer Institute, National Heart Institute, Centers for Disease Control, other federal health agencies, and the World Health Organization.

TOBY CITRIN, J.D., had a background in law and business when he began a second career in public health through an appointment to Detroit's Board of Health in 1969. Since that time, he has steadily augmented his public health activities, serving on a number of appointed state and local health planning, public health, hospital, and health project boards and commissions. During 1974 to 1978, he chaired the Governors Commission to write Michigan's first Public Health Code. He is currently on the faculty of the University of Michigan's School of Public Health, serving as Adjunct Professor of Public Health Policy and Administration and as Executive Director of the school's new Resource for Public Health Policy.

WILLIAM R. ELSEA, M.D., M.P.H., has been Epidemic Intelligence Service Officer, National Centers for Disease Control; Peace Corps Physician; Deputy Commissioner in Buffalo; Health Director for Lexington, Ky., and Cincinnati, Ohio; and President of the National Association of County Health Officials and of the American Association of Public Health Physicians. For the past 12 years he has been Health Commissioner, Fulton County, Atlanta, Ga., and Professor of Community Health, Emory University Medical School.

JOHN R. EVANS, M.D., D. PHIL., is Chairman and Chief Executive Officer of Allelix Inc., a Canadian biotechnology research and development company active in the fields of health and agriculture. He was founding Dean of the Faculty of Medicine and Vice President of Health Sciences at

McMaster University in Hamilton from 1965 to 1972. He served as President of the University of Toronto from 1972 to 1978 and subsequently as Director of the Population, Health and Nutrition Department of the World Bank from 1979 to 1983. Dr. Evans is Director of a number of Canadian corporations and serves as Chairman of the Board of Trustees of the Rockefeller Foundation.

MELVIN M. GRUMBACH, M.D., is the Edward B. Shaw Professor of Pediatrics at the University of California, San Francisco; for more than 20 years he served as Chairman of the Department of Pediatrics. Dr. Grumbach has served on NIH Study Sections, the Board of Scientific Counselors, National Institute of Child Health and Human Development, the General Clinical Research Centers Committee, the NIH Advisory Committee for the Evaluation of Endocrinology and Metabolic Diseases, and the Director's Committee for the Review of the NIH Clinical Center. He was a member of Project Future: Task Force on Academic Child Psychiatry, American Academy of Child Psychiatry. Dr. Grumbach is Past-President of the Association of Medical School Pediatric Department Chairmen, the Endocrine Society, the Western Society for Pediatric Research, and the Lawson Wilkins Pediatric Endocrine Society. He currently is President of the International Pediatric Research Foundation and a member of the International Scientific Council, Foundation Princesse Marie-Christine, Belgium; the Scientific Advisory Board, University of Michigan Center for Human Growth and Development; the Scientific Advisory Board, Hospital for Sick Children, Toronto; the Extramural Review Group, Childrens' Hospital of Los Angeles; and the Institute of Medicine. He is a recipient of the Joseph Mathes Smith Prize, Columbia University; the Borden Award of the American Academy of Pediatrics; and the Robert H. Williams Distinguished Leadership Award of the Endocrine Society.

ROBERT J. HAGGERTY, M.D., is President of the William T. Grant Foundation, which supports research on the mental health of school age children. He is Clinical Professor of Pediatrics at Cornell University Medical School, where he administers the Robert Wood Johnson Foundation's General Pediatric Academic Development Program. He is editor of *Pediatrics in Review* and member of the Institute of Medicine. He was formerly the Roger I. Lee Professor of Health Services at the Harvard School of Public Health and Chairman of the Department of Health Services (which included Maternal and Child Health Services), and from 1964 to 1975 was Professor and Chairman of the Department of Pediatrics, University of Rochester School of Medicine and Dentistry. His initial faculty experience was at Harvard Medical School and Children's Hospital Medical Center, Boston, Mass., where he developed a training and research program in general pediatrics.

He was President of the American Academy of Pediatrics, 1984–85. He is editor (with M. Green) of *Ambulatory Pediatrics* (now in its third edition).

ROBERT HARMON, M.D., M.P.H., is Director of the Missouri Department of Health and Clinical Professor of Family and Community Medicine at the University of Missouri-Columbia School of Medicine. He serves on the Executive Committees of the American College of Preventive Medicine and Association of State and Territorial Health Officials. He is board certified in preventive medicine and has also completed a residency in internal medicine. He was formerly Director of Public Health in Maricopa County, Ariz., and President of the National Association of County Health Officials.

RUTH KNEE, A.C.S.W., is a Consultant on Long-Term/Mental Health Care. While a Federal Civil Servant (1944–1974), she participated in the development of a number of NIMH and other Public Health Service programs directed toward the expansion of community mental health services, improvement of mental hospitals and institutions for the mentally retarded, the mental health role of health and social welfare agencies, quality assurance and financing of health care, and long-term care policies and programs. She has also been a consultant to several federal agencies and private organizations. As one of the founders of NASW, she has served on numerous committees, councils, task forces, and the National Board. She has been one of the NASW representatives to the Joint Commission on Interprofessional Affairs since it was organized. She was the NASW liaison member of the National Mental Health Advisory Council from 1977 to 1981.

LILLIAN MC CREIGHT, R.N., M.P.H., is Assistant Commissioner and State Director of Public Health Nursing in the South Carolina Department of Health and Environmental Control and Adjunct Professor in the USC School of Public Health. She is Past-President of the Association of State and Territorial Directors of Nursing and represented them in the Consensus Conference on Essentials of Public Health Nursing Practice and Education. She directed South Carolina's search project in Community Long Term Care in its initial year. She is a member of APHA's nominating committee and the National league for Nursing Board of Directors.

BEVERLEE MYERS, M.P.H., served until her death in December 1986 as the Professor and Head of the Division of Health Services of the School of Public Health at the University of California, Los Angeles. She was the Director of the California Department of Health Services from 1978 to 1983 and the Deputy Commissioner for Medical Assistance at the New York State Department of Social Services from 1973 to 1976. Professor Myers also served as the Director of the Office of Planning and Evaluation for the

Assistant Secretary for Health and filled various positions with the U.S. Public Health Service. She was on the Board of Directors with the Alan Guttmacher Institute and with the Western Consortium for Health Professions, a member of the Steering Committee on the American Medical Association's Health Policy Agenda for American People, and a member of the Institute of Medicine. She authored many papers on medical care and public health.

BARBARA ROSENKRANTZ, PH.D., is Professor of History of Science in the Faculty of Arts and Sciences and in the Faculty of Public Health at Harvard University. She is Chairman of the Department of History of Science, a member of the Program of Health Policy and Management, and a member of the Institute of Medicine and the American Academy of Arts and Sciences. She is the author of books and articles on the history of public health, include a widely cited study *Public Health and the State: Changing Views in Massachusetts 1832–1946* (1972); editor for history of the *American Journal of Public Health;* and a member of the editorial board of *Bulletin of the History of Medicine.* She serves on the Executive Council of the American Council of Learned Societies as a delegate from the History of Science Society. Her current research focuses on the contributions of the Commonwealth Fund and other twentieth-century foundations for the improvement of public health and services between the two world wars.

ROBERT J. RUBIN, M.D., is Executive Vice President for Health Affairs and a Director of ICF Incorporated, a Washington-based consulting firm. From 1981 until 1984, Dr. Rubin was the Assistant Secretary for Planning and Evaluation at the Department of Health and Human Services. Prior to joining the government, he was an Associate Professor of Medicine and Assistant Dean at Tufts University. Currently, Dr. Rubin, a board-certified internist and nephrologist, is a Clinical Associate Professor of Medicine at Georgetown University School of Medicine.

LOUISE B. RUSSELL, PH.D., is a Research Professor of Economics at the Institute for Health Care Policy, Rutgers University. Until August 1987, she was a Senior Fellow at the Brookings Institution, where she wrote *Is Prevention Better Than Cure?* (1986) and *Evaluating Preventive Care: Report on a Workshop* (1987). She is a member of the U.S. Preventive Services Task Force and a member of the Institute of Medicine.

HARVEY SLOANE, M.D., is County Judge/Executive for Jefferson County, Ky. He served two terms as Mayor of the city of Louisville—December 1973–November 1977 and January 1982–December 1985. He has served as President of the Kentucky Rural Housing and Development Foundation, worked for the U.S. Public Health Service in Eastern Kentucky's rural Martin County, and also as a volunteer physician in Vietnam. The creator of Louisville's Emergency Medical Service and Director of the Park–DuValle Neighborhood Health Center, Sloane also served with a 1962 Nutritional Survey Team to Malaysia and continues as a Clinical Associate Professor for the Department of Community Health, School of Medicine, at the University of Louisville. He recently established the first AIDS Task Force study group for Kentucky.

HUGH TILSON, M.D., DR. P.H., is the Director, Division of Epidemiology, Information and Surveillance, for the Burroughs Wellcome Co., where he has presided over a program of public health services inside the pharmaceutical industry since 1981. From 1972 to 1979, he served as Local Health Officer and Director of Human Services for Multnomah County (including Portland), Oreg., where he created "Project Health," a national model for pooled medical care financing for public clients. From 1979 to 1981, he served as State Health Officer for North Carolina. He has served on clinical and adjunct faculties at the University of Oregon, Duke University, and University of North Carolina, where he is currently Adjunct Professor in the Schools of Medicine, Public Health, and Pharmacy. Dr. Tilson is Past-President of the National Association of County Health Officials and has served for many years as a consultant to the ongoing efforts of colleagues in official state, local, and national public health organizations for Model Standards for Community Preventive Health Services. He is currently feature editor for "Notes From the Field" for the *American Journal of Public Health*. He is currently a trustee of the American Board of Preventive Medicine.

REPRESENTATIVE SARA M. TOWNSEND was elected to the New Hampshire House in 1970. Since then she has served in various leadership positions, including 6 years as Majority Whip. Known as a health care activist, her efforts in legislation have resulted in laws on health care and elderly matters. She is a member of the New Hampshire Task Force on Long Term Care and the Alzheimer's Study Committee. Rep. Townsend is on the Board of Directors of the National Council on the Aging and is concluding 3 years as a member of the Executive Committee of the National Conference of State Legislatures.

BAILUS WALKER, JR., PH.D., M.P.H., is Professor of Environmental Health and Toxicology at the Graduate School of Public Health Sciences, State University of New York at Albany. From 1983 until 1987, he was Commissioner of Public Health and Chairman of the Public Health Council of the Commonwealth of Massachusetts. Prior to that he was State Director of Public Health for Michigan. He has taught at the Harvard School of Public Health and the University of Michigan. He was formerly Director of the Occupational Health Standards Directorate of the U.S. Department of Labor, where he developed the nation's first policy of the identification and communication of hazardous substance information in the workplace. In 1979 he received the Browning Prize for Disease Prevention for his work in reducing the risk of environmentally provoked diseases in urban centers of the United States. He is President of the American Public Health Association and is author of *Occupational Health Problems Faced by Minority Workers*.

J. JEROME WILDGEN, M.D., is, and has been, in private practice since 1955 in Kalispell, Mont. From 1970 to the present he has been a Clinical Instructor at the University of Washington School of Medicine in Family Practice. He was President of the American Academy of Family Physicians in 1971–72, on the Council of Medical Education of the American Medical Association from 1974 to 1981, and Vice President of the American Board of Family Practice in 1976. He has been a member of the Institute of Medicine since 1973.

C

Model Standards

Program Areas

Administration and Supporting
Services
Aging and Dependent Populations
Air Quality
Alcohol and Drug Abuse and
Addiction
Chronic Disease Control
Communicable Disease Control
Immunization
Sexually Transmitted Diseases
Tuberculosis
Dental Health
Emergency Medical Services
Epidemiology and Surveillance
Family Planning
Food Protection
Genetic Disease Control
Health Education
Home Health Services
Housing Services
Injury Control
Institutional Services
Laboratory Services

Maternal and Child Health
Mental Health
Noise Control
Nutrition Services
Occupational Safety and Health
Primary Care
Radiological Health
Sanitation in Facilities
Child Care Facilities
Government and Non-Govern-
ment Public Buildings
Mobile Home Parks
Recreational Areas
Schools
School Health
Solid Waste Management
Tobacco Use and Addiction
Toxic and Hazardous Substances
Vector and Animal Control
Violent and Abusive Behavior
Wastewater Management
Water (Safe Drinking)

Promoting Health/Preventing Disease:
Objectives for the Nation—1990

Preventive Health Services
  High Blood Pressure Control
  Family Planning
  Pregnancy and Infant Health
  Immunization
  Sexually Transmitted Diseases
Health Protection
  Toxic Agent Control
  Occupational Safety and Health
  Accident Prevention and Injury
    Control

  Fluoridation and Dental Health
  Surveillance and Control of In-
    fectious Diseases
Health Promotion
  Smoking and Health
  Misuse of Alcohol and Drugs
  Nutrition
  Physical Fitness and Exercise
  Control of Stress and Violent
    Behavior

D

Site Visits:
Site Selection and Methodology

OBJECTIVES FOR THE SITE VISITS

Site visits to six states were included in the study plan in order to augment the information available to the committee about the current state of public health activities in the United States. The site visits were intended to elicit directly the perceptions of key actors who shape public health activities either through direct participation in those activities or through influence in the establishment of public health policies. The visits were conceived as an opportunity to learn more about the actual functioning of public health in addressing health problems—eliciting information that goes beyond formal organizational statements to probe more deeply into decision processes. This information would add to the committee's understanding of how policies are established and implemented and what problems are encountered that inhibit effective actions.

SITE SELECTION

The selection criteria aimed at a purposive sample that would maximize the opportunities for the committee to learn from visits to only six states—a constraint imposed by time and resources. A purposive sample was viewed by the committee as much more useful and valid than any attempt at randomization with such small numbers. The site visit information would augment other data available to the committee about all states (e.g., the data from the Public Health Foundation), statements at the four regional meetings, and the extensive knowledge and experience of the committee, including detailed knowledge among the committee of 13 additional states.

The selection process sought variety across the following dimensions:

- proportion of urban and rural population
- strength of economy, principal economic activities, and tax base
- intensity of public health activities (absolute and per capita expenditures)
- range of public health activities
- structure of government for public health (e.g., inclusion of public health in "superagency" versus independent public health agency)
- relative roles of state and local government in public health
- continuity of public health leadership

The intention was to visit localities within each state selected as well as the state capital. Therefore, additional opportunity was provided in the selection to represent diversity over these dimensions.

Data and other information on all the states were compiled by staff for consideration by the committee. In addition to the above dimensions, the intent was to choose states to the extent possible where the committee members were not currently active in administration of public health activities.

The final choices were made by the committee. The sites selected included the capitals and several local areas in each of the following states: West Virginia, New Jersey, California, Mississippi, South Dakota, and Washington.

METHODOLOGY

The design of the site visits drew on the recent literature concerned with policy implementation research. (Pressman and Wildavskey, 1973; Nakamura and Smallwood, 1980; Sabatier and Nasmanian, 1980; Tooner, 1985; Williams, 1980) The emphasis of this research is on the transformation, within an administrative system, of inputs (laws, funds, personnel, techniques) into outputs (people served, regulatory activities performed, transfer payments made), and outcomes (lower infant mortality rate, control of infectious disease outbreaks, etc.). The effort is directed toward understanding what is actually going on at the day-to-day operational level of public problem-processing.

The site visits lasted 4 or 5 days. An advance visit was made by staff to arrange the visits. Committee and staff participated in each visit. Descriptive data on each state and locality were distributed to site visitors in advance. Interviewees were selected through interaction with informed persons in each state and locality visited. Interviewees included:

• public health officials (state and local and various levels within each organization)
• officials of related agencies (welfare, environment, Medicaid, etc.)
• elected officials (state and local)
• staff at general purpose government levels (budget officials)
• practicing physicians and nurses
• other health leaders in the private sector (hospital associations, nursing associations, social worker associations)
• consumer leaders
• media representatives

The interview process was semistructured. An interview guide was provided to each interviewer outlining objectives, emphasizing the need to elicit the perceptions of those being interviewed without prejudgment from the interviewer, giving examples of interview techniques to help achieve this purpose and sample questions. The questions were aimed at eliciting not only description and evaluation but also hopes and aspirations for public health. Many of the questions were open-ended rather than highly structured in order to assure that the interviewees' perceptions were guiding the discussion.

A document describing the study and the purpose of the site visits was sent in advance to interviewees. That document outlined a series of nine specific health problems agreed to in advance by the committee in order to provide some initial focus for the interviews. Those problems were:

AIDS	Pertussis Vaccine
Tobacco Use and Addiction	Alzheimer's Disease
Unintended Injuries	Medical Indigence
Hazardous Waste Disposal	Teen-Age Pregnancy
Exposure to Asbestos	

The problem list was used as a starting point. The interviews did not attempt to confine the dimensions to those problems. (Indeed, some interviewees were quite forceful in adding other problems to the discussion.)

Each interviewer wrote up the interviews immediately following the interviews. A summary report on each visit was prepared by staff for the use of the full committee. As confidentiality was promised to interviewees, those reports will not be published. Information from all interviewees was classified by topic and entered into a computer system for later retrieval and analysis.

A shorter visit was made to the health department in Toronto, Canada. This 1-day visit did not follow the process described above, but was intended to provide some additional perspective on public health issues as seen from another political, social, and cultural context. Substantial information on public health activities in Toronto and Ontario was provided to the committee.

REFERENCES

Nakamura, Robert T., and F. Smallwood. 1980. *The Politics of Policy Implementation.* St. Martin's Press, New York.

Pressman, Jeffrey L., and A. Wildavskey. 1973. *Implementation.* University of California Press, Berkeley.

Sabatier, Paul, and R. Nasmanian, eds. 1980. Special Issue on Implementation. *Policy Studies Journal,* vol. 19.

Tooner, Theo A. J. 1985. *Implementation Research and Institutional Design: The Quest for Structure.* Martinus Nijhoff, The Netherlands.

Williams, Walter. 1980. *The Implementation Perspective.* University of California Press, Berkeley.

Index